AF259343

Death Resistant

*A common sense guide to live long
and drop dead healthy*

By Michael Ockrim

© 2021 Mighty Oak Athletic, LLC
All rights reserved
eISBN : 000-0-000-00000-0

Published by Mighty Oak Athletic, LLC
P.O. Box 932, Westmont, Illinois, 60559, U.S.A.

The scanning, uploading and distribution of this book via the Internet or via any other means without the permission of the publisher is illegal and punishable by law. Please purchase only authorized electronic editions, and do not participate in or encourage electronic piracy of copyrighted materials. Your support of the author's rights is appreciated.

Version_1.1
MightyOakAthletic.com

"A recent study suggests you do not "inherit" longevity as much as previously believed. Instead, the sum of your habits determines your life span."

-Tom Rath
Eat Move Sleep: How Small Choices Lead to Big Changes

TABLE OF CONTENTS

PROLOGUE

Recovery, Movement, and Nutrition. That is what it takes to live a long and healthy life. This is not groundbreaking information. Most people intuitively know this to be true. The challenge arises in defining how often, how much, when, where, and what "healthy" rest, activity, and food look like.

The Circles of Life are an attempt to break "healthy" down into manageable segments that can be understood and applied. The goal is not to process all of the information in one sitting and then assimilate that into tomorrow's daily activities.

Rather, start by understanding a high level overview. Grasp the system from a more general point-of-view. Then, gradually begin to break down the individual components and implement them into a personalized definition of "health."

Reserve the right to change as new information becomes available. Health and fitness has evolved for millennia. What is a best practice today, might be completely reversed next year. Do not let that fluidity of thought undermine the mindset as a whole.

Commitment to a healthy and active lifestyle is a life-long journey. Play the long game. Start thinking in terms of living to be 120 years old and what it will take to get there with a sharp mind and a functional body.

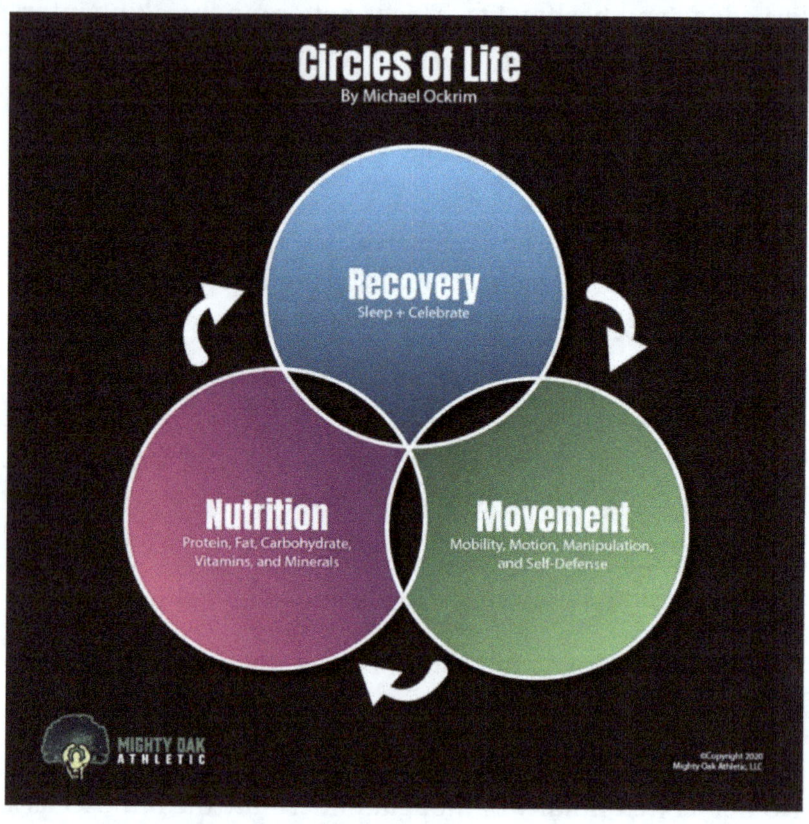

Circles of Life
By Michael Ockrim
Recovery
Sleep + Celebrate
Nutrition
Protein, Fat, Carbohydrate,
Vitamins, and Minerals
Movement
Mobility, Motion, Manipulation,
and Self-Defense
MIGHTY OAK
ATHLETIC
©Copyright 2020
Mighty Oak Athletic, LLC

CIRCLES OF LIFE

Recovery is the most underrated aspect of health. While recovery has been more popular in recent fitness discussions, diet and exercise still dominate the health mindset. This is a mistake. Rest and recovery is where the magic happens. During intense activity, the body gets broken down. Physical growth takes place long after the sweat has dried.

Many people in a pursuit of health tend to over-exercise and under-eat. The common mantra is *eat less and exercise more*. Frustration sets in when the body refuses to respond with the desired effect, or worse, an adverse effect!

So what is the solution? Prioritize rejuvenation. Mighty Oak Athletic will demystify what recovery looks like in the following chapters.

"Rest and recovery is where the magic happens."

Movement

This is the most overrated aspect of health. Ready for the dirty little secret of personal trainers everywhere? One cannot out-train poor nutrition. Exercise is not a means to weight loss.

Exercise needs to be reframed as movement. Which movements build a strong, supple, and useful body? Which movements are essential for a long and healthy life? It is time to ditch the fancy contraptions and joint crushing weights. Embrace natural body motions that support strong bones and muscles, preserve joints and tendons, and progress through a natural range of movement.

Healthy movements improve mobility, build muscular strength, and increase cardiovascular endurance. They also need to be enjoyable. Not all movements will be anxiously anticipated prior to a movement session, but all movements should serve the end goal of an increased *health span* - the part of life when someone is generally in good health. Ditch the exercise mindset and reframe movement into a physical expression of human movement that will improve quality of life for decades to come.

> *"Embrace natural body motions that support strong bones and muscles, preserve joints and tendons, and progress through a natural range of motion."*

Nutrition

This is the most appropriately rated aspect of health. For many years, nutrition information was disseminated primarily by government agencies that, while not necessarily nefarious organizations, had multiple desired outcomes competing for support.

Is a diet based largely on the consumption of grains healthy or the work of large corporations supporting research that built the case for the sale of their products? Is fat the enemy? Maybe some types of fat. What about cholesterol? Is cholesterol found in food the same as cholesterol found in the human body? Thirty years ago, it was challenging to get good information. Today, the opposite challenge has prevailed - too much information. This often leads to paralysis by analysis.

Mighty Oak Athletic will break nutrition down into its basic elements. Then one can begin to understand what is important, what is irrelevant, and what it all means within the scope of a long and healthy life.

Join the conversation by subscribing to the free weekly newsletter at MightyOakAthletic.com

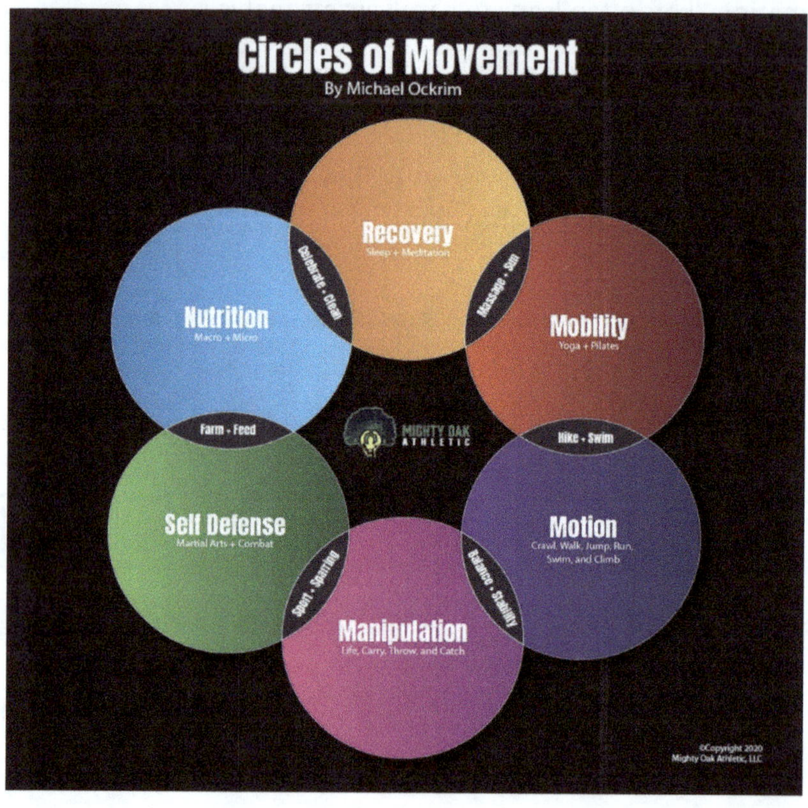
Circles of Movement
By Michael Ockrim
Recovery
Sleep + Meditation
Nutrition
Macro + Micro
Mobility
Yoga + Pilates
Celebrate • Clean
Massage • Sun
Farm • Feed
Hike • Swim
MIGHTY OAK
ATHLETIC
Self Defense
Martial Arts + Combat
Motion
Crawl, Walk, Jump, Run,
Swim, and Climb
Sport • Sparring
Agility • Stability
Manipulation
Lift, Carry, Throw, and Catch
©Copyright 2020
Mighty Oak Athletic, LLC

CIRCLES OF MOVEMENT

What does it take to move well? It requires a shift in thinking and a shift in the approach to fitness.

For thousands of years, mankind had to adapt to their environment. The rapid advancement of technologies in recent centuries has enabled mankind to adapt their environment to them. Earlier versions of humans had to efficiently crawl, walk, run, balance, jump, climb, carry, throw, catch, and defend themselves. These skills were essential for survival in the often unforgiving world around them. Challenges were everywhere!

In modern times, the focus has shifted from being fit for practical reasons to being fit to simply look good. Developing a body that functions well will result in a body that looks great. Muscles will develop naturally and in a symmetrical manner - think Michelangelo's David. More importantly, the body feels well and will handle activities in our daily lives pain-free.

"Developing a body that functions well will result in a body that looks great."

The current approach to fitness is working out on some sort of man-made contraption for 60 minutes a day, three days a week. Then being primarily sedentary for the next 23 hours moving from chairs, to cars, to couches, to beds. People view working out as work, not fun. Movement should be an enjoyable part of life that is peppered in throughout the day.

When "working out," think about how the body moves naturally. Do not default to the man-made machines that tout fitness. Just move. Run. Jump. Carry. Crawl. Throw. Catch. Push something heavy. Pull something awkward. Squat down. Push up. Be creative. Make it a game. Have fun!

Remember, the fitness industry is a business that needs products to sell. There is no way to monetize a pull up...voila!...the lat pull down machine. Ask the fundamental question, has there ever been a time the environment dictated that someone move in the restricted motions of the lat pull down machine - seated, legs immobilized, pulling weight down onto the body?

Food for thought... Now get up and get moving!

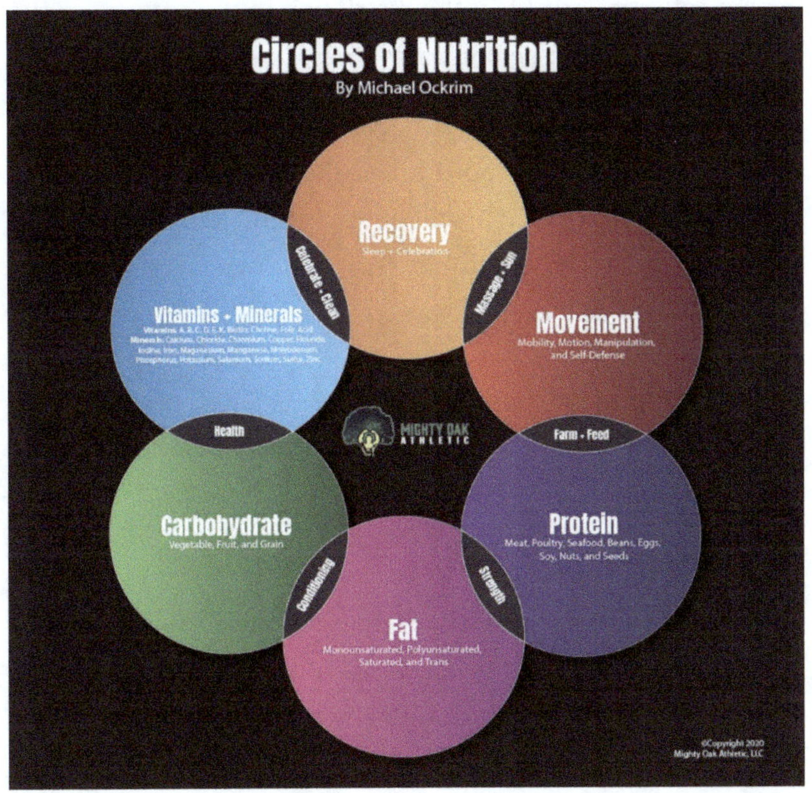
Circles of Nutrition
By Michael Ockrim
Recovery
Sleep + Celebration
Movement
Mobility, Motion, Manipulation, and Self Defense
Vitamins + Minerals
Vitamins: A, B, C, D, E, K, Biotin, Choline, Folic Acid
Minerals: Calcium, Chloride, Chromium, Copper, Fluoride, Iodine, Iron, Magnesium, Manganese, Molybdenum, Phosphorus, Potassium, Selenium, Sodium, Sulfur, Zinc
Carbohydrate
Vegetable, Fruit, and Grain
Protein
Meat, Poultry, Seafood, Beans, Eggs, Soy, Nuts, and Seeds
Fat
Monounsaturated, Polyunsaturated, Saturated, and Trans
Celebrate + Clean
Massage + Sun
Farm + Feed
Strength
Conditioning
Health
MIGHTY OAK ATHLETIC
©Copyright 2020
Mighty Oak Athletic, LLC

CIRCLES OF NUTRITION

Diet. What does that word mean? Is it the types of foods that a person eats regularly? Is it the restriction in the amount or the types of foods that a person eats? Does it matter?

Forget diet. Think nutrition. Nutrition is all about consuming the highest quality foods for health and growth. How nutrition is put into practice will be varied for every person, but some aspects will be consistent regardless of age, race, gender, physical needs, and mental state.

"Nutrition is all about consuming the highest quality foods for health and growth"

Health Savings Account

When making a food or beverage selection, ask the fundamental question: is this going to be a deposit into the health savings account, or a withdrawal. Not all food and beverage selections need to be a deposit, but the ledger needs to stay in the positive.

The adverse effects on health start to arise when the account balance is consistently in the negative - too many withdrawals and too few deposits. That does not mean that the goal is to only make deposits and live a life void of enjoyment. It cannot, however, be strictly focused on hedonistic consumption that keeps making withdrawals long after the account balance has gone negative. When this happens, the body will impose penalties in the forms of mental fatigue, physical discomfort, joint inflammation, weight gain, muscle loss, weakening in the bones, wrinkles in the face…the list goes on and on.

Keep the health savings account analogy top of mind when making food and beverage selections. It is not something to be obsessed about, but rather, to be mindful of. Do not get into the habit of eating without thinking. Be aware of the choices that are being made and acknowledge that there is freedom of choice, but not freedom from consequence.

By consistently choosing nutritious foods that will add to the balance in the health savings account, the ledger will steadily grow, allowing plenty of positive accumulation that can be withdrawn against to enjoy life's culinary pleasures.

"When making a food or beverage selection, ask the fundamental question: is this going to be a deposit into the Health Savings Account, or a withdrawal?"

Avoid alcohol

Imbibing in the occasional beer or cocktail is great! But before cracking open a cold brew, or popping that cork, ask the question: Is this drink worth drinking? Is it truly a moment worth celebrating or a special concoction worth consuming, or is this just a mindless drink.

All too often, consuming alcohol is simply ritual or habitual. Work day is done - Miller Time! Friday night - break out the Chardonnay! Sunday Funday - Bloody Mary's all around! Seemingly, most moments in life get rationalized as a reason for breaking out the booze.

Time to ask the scary question: Is someone able to stop drinking, or are they dependent on alcohol for a variety of reasons? Not sure? Try going dry for 30 days. See how it goes. Can't do it? Consider talking with someone about it.

"Before cracking open a cold brew, or popping that cork, ask the question: Is this drink worth drinking?

Drink plenty of water

Most people consume plenty of liquid throughout the day. That isn't the challenge. *What* they are consuming is the problem.

DON'T DRINK SUGAR! This cannot be overstated. When sugar is consumed in a liquid form, it is sent almost immediately to the blood stream, causing a huge spike in blood sugar levels, insulin response, and a rapid rise and crash in energy levels. This is because the sugar is being ingested with any fiber to slow its' digestion. While eating loads of sugar is also a bad idea, drinking sugar is generally a terrible habit.

This isn't limited to pop and sports drinks, either. Most non-water beverages are loaded with sugar. This includes fruit and vegetable juices, coffee and tea, flavored waters, and alcoholic beverages.

Does that mean that someone should only be drinking water? Yes. And no. It's understood that life is about enjoying the things that bring about a feeling of joy and contentment. Many of these sugary beverages do just that.

The key is to have a shift in the mindset regarding these beverages. Sugary drinks are not something to be consumed on a daily basis - just drink water! Include the sugary drinks sparingly throughout the week at appropriate times. Always ask *how much* and *how often* is reasonable to drink?

Just finished a round of golf with friends? Great! Time to enjoy a sports drink. Girls night out? Fun! Break out the mocktails. Enjoying 1-2 sugary drinks a week is reasonable. Any more than that and the negative effects on health begin to outweigh the positive feelings from enjoying the beverage.

"DON'T DRINK SUGAR!"

Eat the rainbow

Most people simply do not eat enough fruits and vegetables. Or they eat the same 3-4 fruits and vegetables without any variety. Fix this by making fruits and vegetables the main focus of a meal, and eat a variety of colors.

Meat and grain dominate the American plate. This is one of the factors that has lead to staggering numbers of obesity and lifestyle-related health issues. Meat and grains can be a part of balanced nutrition, but all to often the meat and grains take up most of the plate, while the vitamins and minerals found in the fruits and veggies are relegated to an insignificant side note on the perimeter of the plate.

When the fruits and veggies do make it onto the plate, they are often drenched in sauces that are loaded with salt, sugar, and fat.

There also tends to be very little variety. Carrots, bananas, apples, avocados…the usual suspects. These are all healthy option! Eating the same foods meal after meal, however, limits the variety in vitamins, minerals, and phytonutrients (the nutritious stuff found in plants) that the body is getting.

Mix it up. Try to eat fruits and vegetables with different colors each day. Monday might be orange carrots and tangerines. Tuesday can be red bell peppers and raspberries. Wednesday, broccoli and green grapes. Not only will the variety improve nutrition and overall health, it will keep healthy eating interesting and less mundane for the taste buds.

*"Make fruits and vegetables the main focus of a meal,
and eat a variety of colors"*

Higher quality = higher nutrition

Healthy Dirt. Healthy Grass. Healthy Cow. Healthy Meat. Healthy Human. When selecting food, it is important to ask the question: "What is it and where does it come from?

Yes, it is a Cool Ranch Dorito from Walmart - and its delicious! But can it be traced back to flora and fauna? And more importantly, what is the journey of the food?

Is meat healthy? Depends. Lean cuts from a healthy, humanely raised animal can be part of a nutritious diet. Heavily marbled cuts of meat from animals force-fed grain, antibiotics, and growth hormones are bad news.

Choose organic fruits and vegetables. This limits the amount of nasty chemicals that are ingested. An apple a day keeps the doctor away - unless that apple is drenched in pesticides.

Eating quality food can be done on a limited budget. And cooking homemade meals is always less expensive than eating out. To get the best return on investment, focus on buying grass fed meat, eggs from free range chickens, dairy from grass fed animals, and always organic when buying the heavily sprayed Dirty Dozen: apples, bell peppers, celery, cherries, grapes, lettuce, nectarines, peaches, pears, potatoes, spinach, and strawberries.

Be a discerning connoisseur of food. Make an effort to understand the journey that food takes from earth, to store, to plate. Be a healthy human!

> *"Make an effort to understand the journey that food takes from earth, to store, to plate"*

No reading

The healthiest foods do not have nutrition labels. A carrot is a carrot - plain and simple. Carrot cake? That has a lot of ingredients, it is highly processed, and most of the nutrition has been stripped out. Any food with a long ingredient list is man-made and should be avoided.

> *"A carrot is a carrot - plain and simple."*

Size matters

What is the proper portion size? This varies from person to person. The best way to gauge a reasonable portion size is to use the hands.

A serving of meat or fish is the size of the palm - this includes the length, width, and depth of the palm.

A serving of vegetables fills two hands cupped together.

A serving of fruit fills one hand cupped.

A serving of grains is the size of a fist.

A serving of cheese and sweets is the size of a thumb.

Use smaller dishes. Avoid giant plates, bowls, and cups that are begging to be filled. When eating out, ask for a to-go box when ordering and place half of the food in the container before eating; restaurants routinely serve large portion sizes.

"Avoid giant plates, bowls, and cups that are begging to be filled."

Pack it up

Not every meal can be consumed in the home. Avoid the temptation to eat in restaurants or allowing hunger to force poor food choices, by packing a homemade lunch and a water bottle when leaving the home for extended periods. Keep a stash of easy to eat snacks in the car or office. This will help to avoid hangry runs to the vending machine or fast food restaurant. Nuts, seeds, granola, and fruit are always quick and easy snack options.

"Pack a homemade lunch and a water bottle when leaving the home for extended periods."

Make meals mindful

Slow down. Enjoy food. Make eating a shared experience.

Avoid slurping meals while driving, at the desk between meetings, or in a rush before heading out the door.

Take time to schedule eating with family and friends. A nourishing meal is not just the food that goes into the body, it is also the shared positive experience with loved ones.

"Slow down. Enjoy food. Make eating a shared experience."

REST AND RECOVERY

Exercise for exercise's sake is overrated. It is important to build a training program by first defining the goal. Start with the end in mind!

Is the goal weight loss? To build strength? Have bigger muscles? Move better? Eliminate pain? Prepare for a sporting event?

Defining the goal is essential to outline the proper plan for achieving the desired outcome. And the proper plan will include ample rest and recovery for the body to adapt and grow. Do not ignore rest and recovery. That is where the magic happens!

Define the goal. Know exactly what needs to be done in the training to achieve that goal. Then be sure to adhere to the plan and allow for the growth and development to happen.

The training is the stressor that disrupts homeostasis and challenges the body to grow stronger and healthier. That growth, however, cannot take place if the body is in a constant state of stress and fatigue.

The body needs time to recover and rebuild. While the desired outcome might be a beach body for the vacation in 3 weeks, the body cannot always adapt in the artificial time constraints imposed on it by calendars and holiday plans.

Build the plan. Stick to the plan. Be patient. Be consistent. And get some rest!

> *"Do not ignore rest and recovery, this is where the magic happens!"*

REST

On the health underrated list is the power of consistent, deep sleep. Many people spend an inordinate amount of time obsessing about the overrated components of health like exercise and supplements. Meanwhile, the facets of health that truly move the needle in an impactful way - proper nutrition from real food and sleeping habits - are often an after thought.

An overwhelming amount of current research shows that sleep is essential to physical and mental health. The harsh reality is that most people are sabotaging their sleep and missing out on all of the health benefits a sound night of zzz's has to offer.

Here are a few ways to improve sleep quality and overall health. Do not try to implement all of these improvements at once. Choose a single habit to change, and make that the keystone habit (the small change that carries over into other aspects of health) to build upon. This incremental progress is less-challenging to maintain for longer periods of time.

"An overwhelming amount of current research shows that sleep is essential tho physical and mental health."

No screens before bed

That means turn down the harsh LED house lights and power off cell phones, tablets, laptops, PCs, backlit eReaders, and the TV one hour before bed.

LED screens and lights emit blue wavelengths that mess with the body's internal clock and natural rhythms - the circadian rhythm. Screen time and exposure to the now ubiquitous LED lights makes it difficult for the body to begin shutting down after sunset.

Opt for a traditional, non-backlit eReader or print books and magazines when reading for bed.

"LED screens and lights emit blue wavelengths that mess with the body's internal clock and natural rhythms - the circadian rhythm."

Be consistent

Go to bed at the same time every night and wake up at the same time every morning. It is best to allow the body to dictate this, as opposed to an alarm clock.

Following a consistent sleep pattern will set the body's internal clock and condition the mind to expect sleep at the same times each night. A key success factor in achieving this is maintaining the same sleep routine on weekends, as well as during the week. While most people cannot go to sleep and wake up at exactly the same time *every*day, the goal is to stick to the routine most days.

*"Go to bed at the same time every night and wake
up at the same time every morning."*

Trust the body

How many hours should someone sleep each night? It depends. Some people can thrive on 5-1/2 hours of sound sleep. Others need a solid 9 hours of shut eye. Listen to the body and acknowledge the feedback it provides.

While it is easy with a quick internet search to find data that will support a range of required sleep anywhere from 4 to 12 hours per night, 8 hours seems to be the most agreed upon middle ground. Allowing the body and mind to recharge for one third of the day is a reasonable and attainable number for most people. Again, think of hours of sleep as deposits into the Health Savings Account.

"Listen to the body and acknowledge the feedback it provides."

Dark and cool

It's not just screens and LED lights that disrupt sound sleep. Light pollution coming in through windows, or lights from clocks and lamps can have similar negative effects.

Invest in quality blinds or drapes for the bedroom that will block out street lights, passing car lights, and early morning sunlight. On a budget? Block external light with tinfoil "blinds" and cover with inexpensive window dressing.

Have the bedroom comfortably cold before sleep. The external body temperature will adjust under the covers and the internal temperature will set to become comfortably cool - not hot and sweaty.

"Invest in quality blinds or drapes for the bedroom that will block out street lights, passing car lights, and early morning sunlight."

Keep it clean

Eliminate clutter in the bed. Sleeping in minimal clothing and blankets will limit tangles and subsequent tossing and turning. Minimize the number of pillows to create space to move freely. And NO PETS IN BED! The true magic is in deep, undisturbed sleep - not how many hours are spent in bed. Uncertain about the quality of sleep? Check out one of the dozens of sleep tools available to track sleep quality. The results might be eye opening!

"Eliminate clutter in the bed."

Sex and rest

Only use the bedroom for sex, sleep, and light reading. That means no digging into textbooks or work decks - keep the desk outside of the bedroom. Do not chat or text on the phone in bed. Avoid the bedroom when arguing with a partner. Keep the bedroom sacred!

Some people have smaller living spaces or studio apartments. The confined spaces make this maxim challenging to achieve. Make an effort to address these non-sex/rest activities at an alternative location. For anyone with a larger living space - no excuses! - make an effort to compartmentalize activities into the appropriate rooms in the house.

"Only use the bedroom for sex, sleep, and light reading."

Say no to drugs

Alcohol, caffeine, and nicotine destroy a good night sleep. While it may seem like passing out is a deep sleep, it is not restorative. This lack of restorative sleep leads to physical and mental fatigue the next day. This begins the sleep-sapping cycle of caffeine to "wake up", not being able to sleep well from ingesting stimulants throughout the day, waking up groggy, and taking more stimulants. Break the cycle!

"Alcohol, caffeine, and nicotine destroy a good night sleep."

Make it a ritual

Have a bedtime routine that signals to the brain it is time to start shutting down. This might be taking a warm shower or bath, brushing the hair and teeth, applying lotions and potions, and then reading non-work or non-school related books. Find the individual habits that work best and make them a ritual.

"Have a bedtime routine that signals to the brain it is time to start shutting down."

Say sayonara to siestas

Avoid naps during the day. If a nap is necessary, keep it short - 20 minutes - and in the early part of the day.

"Avoid naps during the day."

Postpone pee pee

Stop consuming fluids at least one hour before bed time. This will reduce or eliminate night time trips to the bathroom.

"Stop consuming fluids at least one hour before bed time."

No sweat sesh

Keep strenuous physical activity in the evening - including vigorous sex! - to a minimum. An elevated heart rate and excessive hormones that make the body energetic can make it challenging to relax and fall asleep.

> *"Keep strenuous physical activity in the evening*
> *- including vigorous sex! - to a minimum."*

RECOVERY

In addition to deep, consistent sleep, it is important to engage in activities that promote rest and recovery - not just for the body, but also for the mind and spirit.

Stretching

Stretching is a great way to loosen up tight muscles, wake up sleepy tendons, and warm up creaky joints. It can be used as part of a warm up before physical activity, after a movement session to help the body cool down, during the day to keep the body supple between bouts of prolonged sitting, or before a meeting or exam to wake up the brain and get energy flowing.

Stretching does not have to be a complex sequence of coordinated movements. Listen to the body and stretch what is tight. Some days it may be the shoulders and hips from long hours spent slumped over a laptop. Other days it may be the quads and hamstrings from a long run.

Consistently taking time to stretch will keep the body agile and will reduce the chance of injury. It will also improve mobility at the joints, which will enable proper alignment when doing a variety of movements.

Make stretching a habit. Find ways to include just 5-10 minutes a day to stretch what is tight. Stretching is a classic example of doing a little over the long term having a huge impact on overall health and movement.

"Listen to the body and stretch what is tight."

Massage

There is a distinct difference between stretching and relaxing. Stretching is a great way to loosen up tight muscles, wake up sleepy tendons, and warm up creaky joints. Massage is a way to really get deep into the muscle bellies and allow them to relax.

Massage is also beneficial for the mind. It can be challenging to quiet the brain and block out all of the ongoing chatter that seems to be on a constant loop in the background of the mind.

While a massage can seem like an indulgent experience - which it is! - it is also a key piece in the wellness puzzle that will keep the body feeling strong and mobile. Massage does not have to be a weekly activity. Be consistent, not constant. Aim for a restorative massage once per month to keep the muscles loose, the mind calm, and the body functioning well. Indulge - it's worth it!

"Aim for a restorative massage once per month to keep the muscles loose, the mind calm, and the body functioning well."

Fun in the sun

Sunshine is a free and easily accessible source for instant health improvement. While some people have medical conditions that will limit their ability to enjoy the sun, most people can sunbathe in small spurts most days.

Obviously, the sun has it's strongest effects on the body during summer months, or for those people living close to the equator. But that does not mean the only benefits take place during the warmer months.

Aim for at least 10 minutes outdoors in the sun most days. Some days will be friggin' freezing or oppressively hot, but feeling the sunshine will stimulate a cascade of feel good hormones and emotions in the body. The summer sun is a great source of Vitamin D, which is great for building strong bones and boosting immunity. Soak it up!

"Sunshine is a free and easily accessible source
for instant health improvement."

Meditation

Meditation is often associated with hippie-dippy types that enjoy Save the Turtle rallies and a brunches filled with tree bark and water soup. Some meditation is like that! And it can be really enjoyable. Try taking a deep inhale and letting out a soothing OOOOmmmmm on the exhale. Three to four rounds of Om can do wonders to reset an agitated or anxious mind.

However, not all meditation has to be this style. There are plenty of tasks that can become meditative by getting the mind into a calm, auto-pilot state that will serve to quiet the cascade of thoughts that constantly bombard the conscious brain.

These activities will be different for different people. What activities can be meditative? Slicing and dicing food is a repetitive task that can be calming and allow for contemplative introspection. Gardening and yard work also fit into this category. As do cleaning tasks like vacuuming or sweeping. Looking for something less active? Take time to mindfully make tea or coffee, then sit and enjoy it - preferably outdoors - free from digital distractions. Many times people think that they need a cup of coffee or tea to get reinvigorated, when what they truly need is the tea ceremony.

Take time to identify these meditative activities and make time to enjoy them everyday. It does not have to be a task that takes up a large amount of time. Oftentimes, just 10-15 minutes will do the trick.

OOOOOmmmmm!

> *"There are plenty of tasks that can become meditative by getting the mind into a calm, auto-pilot state that will serve to quiet the cascade of thoughts that constantly bombard the conscious brain."*

Clean up

A dirty and cluttered space can wreak havoc on the minds ability to rest and restore. Clutter can affect anxiety levels, sleep, and the ability to focus. Cleaning is a great way to give the body some active rest - a break from more vigorous training while still getting the body moving.

Do not get overwhelmed and try to clean the entire house or office in one day. Keep it simple. Just 10-15 minutes a day; a little effort over the long term. Start by cleaning and organizing a single drawer or countertop. On more ambitious days, tackle a closet or scrub a bathroom. Even on days when energy levels are low, take time to do some light cleaning. Activity tends to fuel more activity, and will get energy levels up without the need for caffeine or other stimulants.

> *"Cleaning is a great way to give the body some active rest - a break from more vigorous training while still getting the body moving."*

Celebrate

Shared positive experiences with loved ones just might be the meaning of life. Do not let the pursuit of a healthy and active lifestyle take away from the social gatherings in life. Being healthy isn't about being perfect. Keep the Health Savings Account analogy in mind.

If the current social circles are not supportive of leading a healthy and active lifestyle, seek out or build an intentional community of like-minded friends and family that enjoy similar healthy pursuits like being active and cooking nutritious food. It does not mean completely ditching the non-healthy group; just find a balance in the time dedicated to both groups and everything will work itself out.

"Being healthy isn't about being perfect."

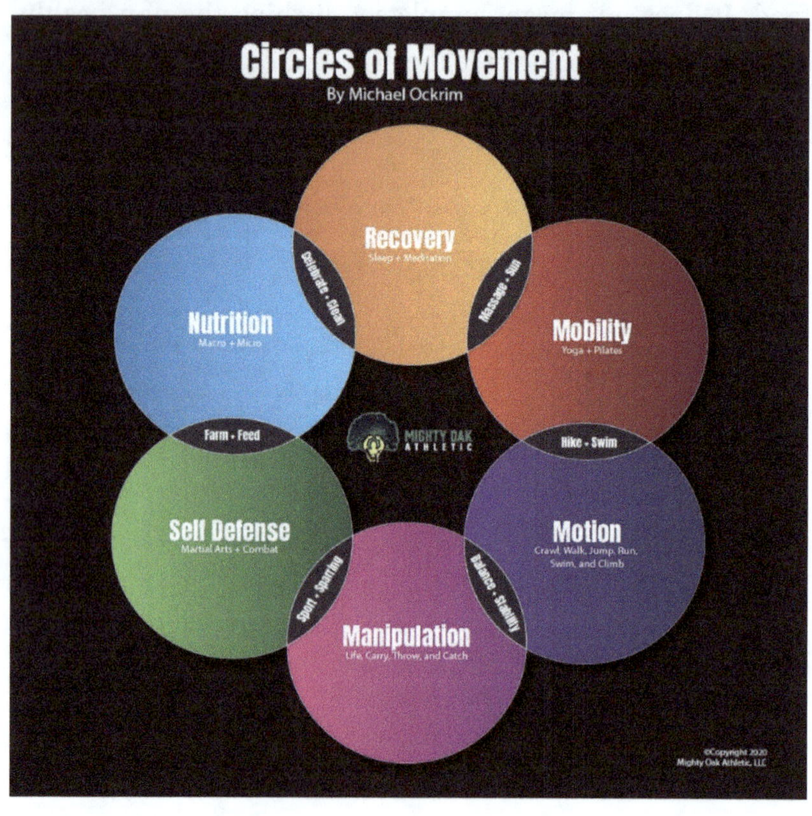
Circles of Movement
By Michael Ockrim
Recovery
Sleep + Meditation
Celebrate + Clean
Massage + Sun
Nutrition
Macro + Micro
Mobility
Yoga + Pilates
Farm + Feed
Hike + Swim
MIGHTY OAK
ATHLETIC
Self Defense
Martial Arts + Combat
Motion
Crawl, Walk, Jump, Run,
Swim, and Climb
Sport + Sparring
Balance + Stability
Manipulation
Life, Carry, Throw, and Catch
©Copyright 2020
Mighty Oak Athletic, LLC

CIRCLES OF MOVEMENT EXPLAINED

A healthy body is mobile, agile, balanced, coordinated, strong, and lean. It can pass through a full range of motion at the joints, move effortless on land and in water, maintain balance on a variety of surfaces, move heavy objects safely and effectively, play sports and participate in games, defend itself in a challenging situation, and perform the basic human movements required for activities in everyday life - squat down, push up, pull up, lift an object off the ground, and carry an object for distance.

Mobility is the key to unlocking healthy movement. Without the ability to move the body through a full range of motion at the joints, everything else will suffer. The body will be forced into adaptive positions to compensate for a poor range of motion, leading to injuries. Make mobility a priority.

An inability to move is one of the biggest indicators of poor health and leads to a shortened health span and lifespan. The less someone moves, the quicker the body and mind deteriorate. Make movement throughout the day - walking - a priority.

Be strong to be useful; and to be able to move the body through the various activities of daily living. Strong legs can get the body in and out of chairs (and off toilets!). A strong core will keep the body stable and free from falls. Strong muscles in the chest and shoulders can place bags in the airplane's overhead storage compartment. A strong back and rump can lift grocery bags and laundry baskets with ease. Make strength a priority.

Humans have had to defend themselves since the beginning of time. It is only recently that society has become significantly less violent. While there is still violence in the world, it is more isolated and concentrated. That does not mean that self-defense should be disregarded as a barbaric endeavor leftover from generations past. Knowing how to safely and effectively defend oneself builds a quiet confidence that will deter the muggers, buggers, and thieves. Make self-defense a priority.

The following sections take a deeper dive into the concepts of mobility, motion, manipulation, and self-defense, and detail how to effectively incorporate them into a healthy and active lifestyle.

"A healthy body is mobile, agile, balanced, coordinated, strong, and lean."

MOBILITY

Movement starts with mobility - the body's ability to move freely and easily.

Good Mobility = Good Movement Patterns = Less Injury = Ability to Move = Good Health

Without a healthy, full range of motion, the body cannot function at it's best. Limited mobility leads to a limited range of motion. When the motions of the body are restricted, injuries occur as the body compensates and moves in inefficient ways. When the body is injured, overall movement will decrease. Lack of movement leads to a decline in health.

Strength and conditioning get all of the attention. Fitness enthusiasts and weekend warriors alike tend to focus on physical efforts like lifting weights, running, biking, and swimming. Mobility is often relegated to a few half-hearted quadriceps or hamstring stretches before diving right into training.

This is a mistake! Mobility improves movement patterns and range of motion. This will improve performance and decrease injuries through better quality of movement, improved control trough a full range of motion, and increased speed of movement with control. Mobility in the hips is of utmost importance, whereas stability is most important at the knee and ankle joints.

Not only should mobility work be included as part of a warm up AND cool down, it also needs to be given a dedicated day in a training schedule. It can take various forms, but generally, mobility training is a yoga or Pilates session.

"Good Mobility = Good Movement Patterns = Less Injury = Ability to Move = Good Health"

Yoga

Stretchy pants, soccer moms, and hippy-dippy Earth biscuit types are what most people envision when thinking about a yoga practice. This is not inaccurate! That does not mean that yoga cannot be highly beneficial for most people. It requires a beginner's mindset, and the ability to keep the ego in check, in order to honestly assess where the body is at physically and what is needed to improve movement and mobility.

For most people, a simple yoga practice can be a complete game changer in their ability to move well and feel healthy. A simple pose like Down Dog will open up the wrists, forearms, shoulders, hips, hamstrings, calves, and ankles. Putting just a handful of movements into motion - the Sun Salutation - will not only increase flexibility, but improve the body's ability to move in sync as a coordinated unit.

This improvement in flexibility and movement will make it easier to complete basic activities in daily life, and improve performance in most recreational physical activities.

Sign up for a yoga class, check the ego at the door, and embrace the opportunity to gradually improve mobility, agility, flexibility, and full-body movement patterns.

"Sign up for a yoga class, check the ego at the door, and embrace the opportunity to gradually improve mobility, agility, flexibility, and full-body movement patterns."

Pilates

Proper body movements generally start in the center of the body - the core. This requires a balanced development of strength in all of the muscles of the abdomen. Most people focus on the six pack mirror muscles. What is often neglected are the muscles on the side of the abdomen, the lower back, and all of the stabilizing muscles deep in the core.

Pilates is an excellent series of movements to significantly strengthen the muscles of the core. While Pilates can be done using special equipment like the Reformer, it is not required. There are numerous movements that can be done by simply lying on the floor.

Connecting with a coach or taking a mat Pilates class can open the door to a world of core strengthening exercise that will keep the body strong and injury free. It is eye opening how lingering injuries and nagging discomfort can be alleviated by taking the time to systematically strengthen the muscles of the core.

"It is eye opening how lingering injuries and nagging can be alleviated by taking the time to systematically strengthen the muscles of the core."

Hike

Americans spend a staggering 93% of their life indoors - 87% inside buildings and 6% inside automobiles. The 7% spent outdoors adds up to a paltry *half a day per week*!

Embrace the old cliche and take a hike. That's it! Get outside and walk around. While it is preferable to be in nature, just being outdoors is a great start for most people.

Hiking in nature has additional health benefits beyond being outside and moving around. Natural environments - beaches, forests, parks - can quiet the mind, lower stress, and cultivate a sense of connection with the world and community. Two hours a week is the *minimum* each person should spend outdoors in nature.

"Americans spend a staggering 93% of their life indoors."

Swim for mobility

Water is a phenomenal training tool to improve mobility and alleviate the stress of gravity on cranky joints and tender muscles. Being a strong swimmer is not required to make use of water as a mobility tool.

Walking in water is a great way to rehab from a lower body injury and allow the body to move in a gentle way. The level of difficulty can be increased by simply increasing the speed at which the movement is completed. High-level athletes run, jump, and shuffle in the water to improve strength by using the steady resistance of the water.

There are also numerous tools that can be used to aid in water training. Grab a kick board to immobilize the arms and build strength in the hips and legs. Or squeeze a foam block between the knees to work on shoulder strength and upper body mobility.

Do not be intimidated to get in the water. Start shallow and use this amazing tool as a secret weapon to improve mobility and build overall physical strength.

"Water is a phenomenal training tool to improve mobility and alleviate the stress of gravity on cranky joints and tender muscles."

MOTION

Strength is easier to develop than many of the other aspects of physical ability. As a result, most people focus their training efforts on getting stronger and building muscle, and less effort focused on other movements that improve balance, coordination, speed, and agility. Improving these other skills would put their strength to greater use in daily life, as well in recreational activities.

Crawl

Humans crawl before they walk. It is a foundational movement pattern that is innate for all people. Very few people, however, crawl after they grow up and stop playing. This is a huge mistake!

Make crawling a part of any balanced movement practice. Crawls can be done during warm up, as a strength and conditioning workout, or as a way to supplement other training exercises.

There are dozens of crawling variations. Start with the basic hand and foot (leopard) crawl moving forward and backward. Move up to inverted (crab walk) crawls and side ways (monkey) crawls. Make crawling fun and move in ways that feel natural. There is no right or wrong answer!

"Humans crawl before they walk."

Walk

Take a walk. Around the house, around the block, or around the park. Walking is one of the most basic of all human movements. A person's overall health can often be predicted simply by looking at how freely and easily they are able to walk.

Walking is an activity that should be done throughout the day, everyday, without exception. Humans are built to walk. The current trend is to track steps. This can be a great way to bring awareness to movement, but a walking practice does not need to be that complicated. Just stand up and walk around!

Be consistent, not constant. Walking a little bit everyday will have a larger return on overall health than walking for longer stretches in more sporadic bursts throughout the month.

In addition to the physical benefits of walking, getting up and moving is a great way to clear the mind and give the brain the space it needs to relax and solve complex problems.

Walking in nature also serves to calm the mind and alleviate stress in the brain by eliminating many of the man-made distractions that act as stressors for the head. Leave the phone at home, take out the ear buds, and get immersed in the sights and sounds of the natural world.

"Walking is an activity that should be done throughout the day, everyday, without exception."

Run

Humans' ability to run at a slow pace over long distances is one of the things that sets them apart from the majority of the animal kingdom. Running is a natural movement, that when done with proper technique, and in moderation, can be a healthy activity.

The challenge for many people is that their technique is causing them pain (excessive heel striking!), or that the volume that they are running is causing overuse injuries.

The mantra: a little over the long term, should absolutely be applied to running. Getting out for a leisurely jog once or twice a week is great. Grinding out miles on the pavement everyday can wreak havoc on the ankle, knee, and hip joints.

To ensure proper running technique, connect with a coach to analyze foot strike, stride, and body movement patterns. A few simple modifications can go a long way in injury prevention.

Run on natural surfaces whenever possible. Grass and sand are forgiving on the body. Asphalt and concrete are punishing on the joints.

Barefoot walking and running are best. There are a few caveats, however. First, only go barefoot on natural surfaces - grass, dirt, sand - no roads or sidewalks. Second, start by walking barefoot to get the feet accustomed to all of the feedback the ground is providing. Next, start by running backwards to force the proper foot strike pattern - landing on the fore foot. Finally, build up the distance gradually. Used to running 3-5 miles in shoes? Start with a half mile barefoot, then lace up the sneakers to finish the run.

While slow, long distance running is beneficial, sprinting can be a physical game changer for most people. Again, build up gradually. Take time to warm up properly with a short walk and light jogging. Then, start with short (10-20 yard) runs at three quarters of maximum speed. Gradually increase the speed and distance as the body adapts to the more intense movement.

"Running is a natural movement, that when done with proper technique, and in moderation, can be a healthy activity."

Jump

Snake! This is the moment where the person leaps out of striking distance from the fangs. Or how about taking a hike and needing to get across a small stream without getting the shoes soaked.

The ability to jump over and across things is an important human movement that many people simply cannot do effectively. It is often due to a lack of practice.

Jumping is easy to incorporate into an existing training routine, or add into activities of daily life. It can even be a workout all on its own!

Walking in a parking lot? Practice jumping over the low cement parking barriers. Jump forward and backward; side to side; zig zag. Try to jump on top and land without losing balance. Balance on top and try to jump to the end of the parking space. There are all sorts of varieties and combinations that can be done.

Working on strengthening the legs with squats or deadlifts? Add in a few jumps up onto a bench at the end of the training. Out for a jog? Practice jumping line-to-line on the sidewalk.

Jump with one foot or two feet; land on one foot or two feet. Alternate feet Olympic triple jump style. Run on the beach and leap forward Olympic long jump style. Break out an old mattress and go for a Fosbury Flop!

The ability to jump and land efficiently, like a cat, has become a lost art. Regain the ability to move like a supple panther by practicing jumping consistently and in a variety of ways.

> *"Regain the ability to move like a supple panther by practicing jumping consistently and in a variety of ways."*

Climb

Climbing trees is for kids. Sure. Climbing is also a fundamental human movement that has been used for survival since the early days of humans. Being a proficient climber - the ability to get the body up and over an object - can be critical in getting out of harms way, and builds a body that functions effectively and efficiently.

Out of climbing practice? Start simple by incorporating the arms and legs in a basic coordinated pattern, like climbing ladder. Progress to more complex variations like climbing low tree branches that require a similar arm and leg movement pattern, but have the "rungs" placed at varying heights and distances. Move on to more complex variations like pulling onto a tree branch with the arms, then swinging the legs up and on top.

Climbing can require the use of a lot of upper body pulling strength. Build up the pulling muscles by practicing hanging from a bar or tree branch; jumping up to get the chin above a bar or branch and then lowering down under control; or by doing pull ups and chin ups.

"Being a proficient climber - being able to get the body up and over an object - can be critical in getting out of harms way, and builds a body that functions effectively and efficiently."

Swim

Of all the aspects of movement, the ability to swim is the one that will most likely save someone's life. Swimming has numerous health benefits like building muscular strength, improving cardiovascular conditioning, loosening joints and improving mobility. Swimming, however, is first and foremost a life skill.

Being comfortable submerged in water takes time. Start at a pool in the shallow water. Practice basic freestyle and breast-stroke. Use flotation devices like kick boards and leg bolsters to assist with isolating movements for the legs or upper body. Spend time floating on the back while breathing calmly and allowing the water to support the body.

Gradually move up to swimming in open bodies of water. Opt for locations with sandy beaches that have calm inlets with gentle waves and lifeguards on duty. This allows for a gradual progression into deeper water

Swimming is a phenomenal total body workout that will improve almost all of the body's physical functions. Embrace the challenge of overcoming the fears associated with water. The time committed to learning how to swim will have a huge return on investment. And just might save a life!

"Swimming is a phenomenal total body workout that will improve almost all of the body's physical functions."

Balance

Whether it is to perform at a high level in sports or to simply keep from falling and breaking a hip, balance is an oft neglected aspect of movement. Balance is the body's ability to stay upright and steady. Training for balance can be added as part of a training program, or sporadically during daily movement.

Balance comes from the center of the body, start by strengthening the muscles of the core (abdomen). By building a strong and stable core, the body will be better equipped to make adjustments to the constantly changing environment that works to knock the body of balance.

The core is not just the six pack abs! All of the muscles in the front, sides, and lower back of the abdomen need to be strengthened. And not just the muscles that can be seen in the mirror. A balanced core has strong muscles deep in the abdomen that assist with stabilization of the hips and spine.

A great way to begin strengthening the core is to hold a push up position plank. The goal is two minutes, but start with less time and build up. Add in side planks to strengthen the obliques and muscles along the side body. Aim for one minute per side. Finally, lie flat on the stomach and curl up, lifting the hands and feet off of the ground. This movement is commonly referred to as cobra. Cobra strengthens the muscles in the lower and middle back.

Once the core has developed some strength, it is time to add balance-challenging movements into daily activities and into training sessions. An easy way to start is by walking on top of street curbs. The narrow surface will work on challenging the body to stay upright without stepping off into the street or grass. Obviously, this needs to be done on streets without a lot of cars. No one should do balance training while dodging oncoming traffic!

*"Whether it is to perform at a high level in sports or
to simply keep from falling and braking a hip, balance is
an oft neglected aspect of movement."*

Stability

Weakening of muscles around the the ankle, knee, and hip joints can lead to a lack of stability in the body. This is what people are referring to when they say a knee buckled or a leg gave out. While weak muscles at the joints are not the only cause for a loss of stability, it is the most common of the culprits. To rebuild strength at the joints, start by moving the joints.

To strengthen ankles, start by sitting in a chair and placing bare feet on the ground. Then slowly lift the heels, alternating feet, pressing into the ball of the foot. Next, move the feet out, creating a 45 degree angle at the knee. Press the heel into the ground and lift the toes up and off of the ground. Again, alternate feet. Now stand up. Balance on one leg (if you are unable to do this, talk with your doctor!) and make large circle in the air with the big toe. Work clockwise and counter-clockwise. Switch feet.

Weak knees can be strengthened in a variety of ways. Start by sitting in a chair with the feet flat on the ground. Flex the right leg to raise the foot straight out. Squeeze the muscles around the knee when the leg is flexed. Alternate legs. Now stand up. Squat down, lowering the rump to the chair - do not sit down - then stand back up. Use a sturdy chair to land safely on the rump if it becomes too difficult to stand up. If this movement is not possible, practice squatting by holding onto a fixed object like a doorway or pole, sit low, and use the arms to help pull back up to standing.

Healthy hips work efficiently when the body moves side-to-side. Start with simple side steps in both directions. Build up to more dynamic movements like shuffles, grapevines, or skaters. Another hip strengthening movement is high stepping. Set up a low object like a water bottle, and practice stepping over the bottle, side-to-side, in both directions.

Build stable joints. It will keep the body from falling and getting injured. The exercises to build stable joints can be a bit tedious. Don't make these exercises the focal point of a training program. Pepper them in throughout the day when sitting at a desk or waiting on a bench. The time and effort invested in stability work will pay dividends in the later years of life.

"The time and effort invested in stability work will pay dividends in the later years of life."

MANIPULATION

Strength training is generally associated with lifting weights. This is a very narrow view of building strength, and leaves little latitude in designing a well-rounded strength training program as part of a healthy movement program.

Another challenge is that strength training is linked to how much weight a person can move. Increasing measurable strength does not necessarily correlate to improved movement or physical health.

It is useful to reframe strength training as *training for functional strength* - strength that can be applied to daily performance. As an example, using the leg extension machine in a gym will build muscular strength and size in the leg. It will not, however, do much to improve functional strength in the legs.

Functional strength requires a symphony of balance, coordination, and reciprocal muscles working in concert to move the body in an efficient and effective manner. Humans do not jump by simply flexing the knee; they use the hip, knee, and ankle joints to load the legs and spring upward.

Train movements, not muscles. Training muscles in isolation - working from a single joint (e.g. biceps curl) - creates incorrect motor programming and causes confusion for the muscles and the brain. This is because the muscles are asked to do one motion in training, then another motion in life. Muscles work together as part of an integrated unit; they should be trained in a similar manner.

Strength training is a means to an end, not an end itself. Start by developing healthy movement pattens using just bodyweight exercises (i.e. push ups, pull ups, air squats, toe touches). This will develop strength along with the balance, proprioception, and synergistic muscles needed to allow for proper progression and preparation for more challenging resistance.

Another great way to train functional strength is through movements that use multiple joints, in multiple planes of motion like working diagonally and rotationally. Using tools like kettlebells and dumbbells (or medium-sized rocks!) allow for these large, multidirectional/planar movements while working just one side of the body. This will simultaneously improve strength while challenging balanced and stabilization across the body.

"Train movements, not muscles."

Lift

Be strong to be useful. Strength is achieved by moving progressively heavier resistance. This can be bodyweight or an object. The weight is generally lifted by pushing or pulling. Pushing and pulling can take on various forms.

Pulling with the upper body can be as simple as opening a door, or as challenging as a pull up. Pushing can be closing a door, or pressing the body up off of the ground.

Lower body pulls are basic toe touches or lifting an object like a laundry basket off the ground. Lower body pushing motions get the body off of the toilet when moving from seated to standing, or when squatting down and up to grab something on the floor.

These are the basic human movements required for the activities of daily living. When these basic movements deteriorate, people become dependent on others or assistance tools (grab bars, automatic doors). This leads to even less movement and a downward health spiral. It also erodes a person's independence and self-reliance.

Take time everyday to do some basic push and pull lifts. Start gradual and build up to more advanced movements and heavier weights as the body builds strength and coordination. The future person in the mirror will be thankful!

"Be strong to be useful."

Carry

Picking up an object and walking with it for distance is one of the most essential human movements. Very few people make an effort to practice carrying heavy or awkward objects in their training.

Often times, the only time people carry anything is when they absolutely have to. This is why so many people get injured carrying everyday objects like grocery bags and laundry baskets.

Carrying requires not just strength in the primary muscles that are holding the object, but it also requires strength in the small muscles that keep the body balanced and the muscles that work as anti-rotational stabilizers.

This does not mean that an entire training session needs to be dedicated to carrying objects around. First, find ways to carry throughout a training session. It can be as simple as taking weights to and from a rack, lugging equipment to an outdoor training space, or being a good gym goer and racking the plates after use.

Carrying is also a great way to finish up a training session. It can be done carrying an object or a training partner! Maybe grab a kettlebell and swing it for 25 reps, then suitcase carry it in each hand for 20 yards. Or bear hug a training partner and walk holding them up. Feeling particularly strong? Squat down and lift the partner over the shoulder and fireman walk.

Being able to safely and effectively carry objects will lead to a longer and pain-free life. It will also make someone useful if faced with a challenging situation that requires carrying someone to safety. Make carrying a staple in any program or daily movement practice. It does not have to be overly complicated or extensive. Be consistent, not constant, and make carrying heavy and awkward objects a habit.

> *"Being able to safely and effectively carry objects will lead to a longer and pain-free life."*

Throw

Humans should not be the dominant species on the planet. They lack so many of the strengths of other animals - speed and agility of a gazelle, size and strength like a Silverback gorilla, climbing ability of big cats, sharp vision like a hawk that can see small objects hundreds of yards away, a dog's nostrils that work independently to smell in stereo, or rotating horse ears that facilitate 360 degree hearing.

What has set humans apart is their large brain, opposable thumbs, and ability to throw objects with speed and accuracy. The combination of these skills empowered humans to imagine weapons like spears, hold tools to make the spear, and then accurately throw the spear at unsuspecting animals.

Whether it is a ball, frisbee, or beanbag, modern humans mostly throw for fun, not survival. These activities are great for adding variety to an active lifestyle, but they do little to train the body and strengthen the shoulder joints.

Throwing is a great activity to warm up the body and build explosive power in the shoulders and hips. Have fun with it!

Grab a medium-sized rock or medicine ball. Start with a basic chest toss (like in basketball), then practice an overhead toss (like in soccer), hinge and throw overhead (like a strongman competitor), or do a single arm shot put throw (like Hamish in Braveheart).

Throwing can be done with a partner, against a brick wall, or a into sturdy tree trunk (a Mighty Oak!). Start with lighter weight and focus on generating a powerful and explosive movement that works the entire body. This will build up strong and healthy joints in the shoulders, hips, and knees.

"Throwing is a great activity to warm up the body and build explosive power in the shoulders and hips."

Catch

A significant amount of training movements is focused on acceleration (running, jumping, lifting) and deceleration (landing, catching) is often overlooked. An inability to effectively decelerate, and slow the body once in motion, can lead to injury in the form of tears in the ligaments or strains in the muscles.

An effective way to improve deceleration is to train eccentric movements - lengthening a muscle while resisting weight. Catching is an example of this type of training. Find a partner and make catching a part of a throwing practice.

Start by working chest tosses and overhead throws. This works best with softer objects like padded medicine balls. It is also safer to have the object bounce before catching it while building up coordination. As catching skills improve, progress to catching the object in the air.

This training can also be done without a partner. Toss an object against a wall or tree and work on catching it off the rebound. Or deadlift and clean the object from the ground to the chest, squat down, then explode upward and throw it straight up. Watch the object and softly catch it using the shock absorbers across the entire body - the muscles in the arms, torso, and legs, as well as bending at the knees, hips, shoulders, and elbows.

Catch to improve the body's ability to decelerate and stay injury free. Just a few reps at each training session will keep the body strong and agile.

> *"An inability to effectively decelerate and slow the body*
> *once in motion, can lead to injury in the form of tears*
> *in the ligaments or strains in the muscles."*

Sport

Physical activity needs to be enjoyable. What an enjoyable activity is will vary from person-to-person. Sports are a great way to bring friendly competition and gamesmanship into training. Sports are also an opportunity to test one's current strengths and weaknesses.

It is one thing to believe that the body is strong, agile, and athletic; it is another to test it and know for sure. Sports provide a fun and engaging way to assess the body's overall competency and physical abilities.

Not all sports need to be a competition against other competitors. Sometimes the best insights come from solo endeavors like swimming in a lake, hiking up a mountain, or practicing martial arts.

Competing against another person - as an individual or member of a team - adds a layer of cooperation and camaraderie that develop a strong athletic community. Often times, it is the community, not the activity, that makes a sporting event enjoyable. In fact, some sports can be grueling (Spartan Race?!), but the shared experience makes it manageable and maybe even fun!

Participating in sports is also a great way to train and develop the body in a natural way. Many training programs can be repetitive or impractical when applied to everyday life. Most sports, however, use the body as a coordinated unit and improve balance, coordination, agility, and stamina.

Explore new sports. It is great to build up proficiency in a single sport, but being a generalist will develop the body in a more complete manner, as well as limit overuse injuries from repetitive motions.

Sports are also a great mental reprieve from the stresses of daily life. When playing a game, the mind needs to be focused on the task at hand. It cannot be distracted by grocery lists and laundry rotations. Sports require undivided attention. That is a great work out for the mind and the spirit!

"Sports provide a fun and engaging way to assess the body's overall competency and physical abilities."

Sparring

Physical play is seen all across the animal kingdom. It can be two puppies chasing and nipping at each other, or two siblings wrestling in the playroom. This physical outlet is not just natural, it is essential.

Humans need healthy physical contact with other humans. They also need to move their body in a way that can free it from the grasp or attack of another human. Modern society is violence-free for the majority of people the majority of the time. As a result, sparring has been disregarded as a more barbaric activity for cage fighters and street thugs. This is a mistake!

Knowing how to move the body in a way that can free it from danger is an essential human skill. Do not dismiss it as something that only those seeking danger will need to employ. An ability to keep oneself safe builds a deeply rooted confidence that can be sensed by other people.

Take the time to incorporate safe and effective sparring techniques into training. Find a partner, wrestle around, have fun and practice sparring. Not only is sparring a great workout, it just might come in handy one day!

"Knowing how to move the body in a way that can free it from danger is an essential human skill."

SELF DEFENSE

Martial Arts

Martial arts' come in numerous styles and forms. Which style someone practices is less important than being committed to a consistent practice. Find a style that is interesting and pursue it to mastery. It is not about what someone knows, it is what they know well!

In general, the martial arts' styles are striking (Karate, Taekwondo, Kung fu, etc.) or grappling (judo, jujitsu, wrestling, etc.). Striking styles will include both the hands and feet, as well as movements like forms (katas) that improve the shifting of body weight to generate power. Grappling styles can work from both a standing position or on the ground. Grappling focuses on forcing an opponent into a submissive position and, conversely, escaping from a submissive position.

Competency in martial arts equates to self-confidence. Very few trained martial artists end up using their skills in a self defense situation because the confidence and manner in which they carry themselves deters any would-be assailant.

Do not overthink a martial art practice. Find a style that looks appealing, visit a few training facilities, talk with the instructors and students, then commit to the one that feels like the best fit. Do not be intimidated by a lack of experience. Most martial arts facilities are the opposite of what most people perceive - they are a friendly community of welcoming individuals that enjoy the art, not the fight.

"Competency in martial arts equates to self-confidence."

Combat

Combat training includes the more aggressive styles of martial arts like Krav Maga, Hapkido, and Muay Thai. These styles can be an intimidating place to start a martial arts journey. Not because the participants are not kind or welcoming, but because the aggressive nature of the styles often come with more bumps and bruises from the start.

Training the more aggressive side of martial arts better prepares the mind for a physical altercation. These styles desensitizes the body and brain to physical contact by providing a stressful and challenging training environment.

Humans have fought in hand-to-hand combat since forever. It is an essential human skill whether it is socially acceptable or not. Therefore, it should be strongly considered for inclusion in a martial arts practice.

Approach combat training with an open mind. Be honest and open with instructors about any concerns. The majority of combat coaches are soft-spoken, caring individuals that are passionate about their craft and are willing to share it in a way that is appealing to each individual that practices at their studio.

"Humans have fought in hand-to-hand combat since forever."

Farm

Access to food is not a modern concern for most people. Grocery stores and restaurants line the streets of most towns around the world. There is also a proliferation of convenient, highly-processed "food" at every gas station, hardware store, and department store. Food is everywhere!

What has happened is that most people have lost the connection to their food. They cannot explain what their food is and where it came from. Food has become some odd shape, sprinkled with seasoning, and packaged in bright bags. Rarely can someone trace it back to nature or create it in a kitchen.

Reconnect with food. Start small. Even the tiniest apartment can accommodate a small herb garden in the windowsill. This connection to food will make eating a more personal and mindful endeavor. It will also provide a physical activity that will bare literal fruits from the labor.

"Reconnect with food."

Feed

Food isn't just fuel for the body; it is nourishment for the spirit. Cooking is a creative and meditative process that requires focus and can calm a busy mind. Food brings people together and strengthens bonds among families, friends, and strangers.

Do not outsource every meal to a restaurant. Make time to cook. Share that food with others. Enjoy the meal. Make eating a pleasurable experience. Let the kitchen table be the most sacred space in the home. Honor the time spent with friends and family around the table. Shared positive experiences with others just might be the meaning of life!

"Shared positive experiences with others just might be the meaning of life!"

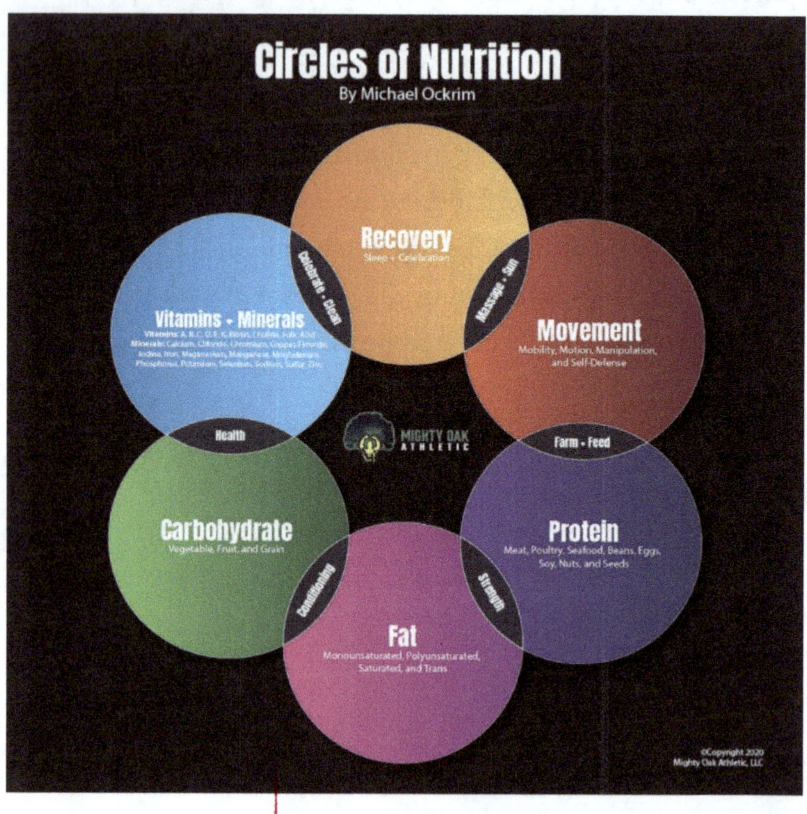
Circles of Nutrition
By Michael Ockrim
Recovery
Sleep + Celebration
Celebrate • Clean
Massage • Sun
Vitamins • Minerals
Vitamins: A, B, C, D, E, K, Biotin, Choline, Folic Acid
Minerals: Calcium, Chloride, Chromium, Copper, Fluoride,
Iodine, Iron, Magnesium, Manganese, Molybdenum,
Phosphorus, Potassium, Selenium, Sodium, Sulfur, Zinc
Movement
Mobility, Motion, Manipulation,
and Self-Defense
Health
Farm • Feed
MIGHTY OAK
ATHLETIC
Carbohydrate
Vegetable, Fruit, and Grain
Protein
Meat, Poultry, Seafood, Beans, Eggs,
Soy, Nuts, and Seeds
Conditioning
Stretch
Fat
Monounsaturated, Polyunsaturated,
Saturated, and Trans
©Copyright 2020
Mighty Oak Athletic, LLC

CIRCLES OF NUTRITION EXPLAINED

At more fruits and vegetables. If there is one message to take away from this book, that is it. Most people eat too few fresh, organic fruits and vegetables. By simply increasing the amount of fruits and vegetables consumed, and subsequently decreasing the amount of other foods eaten, a person can make significant improvements to their health.

Fruits and vegetables fall into the macronutrient category of carbohydrates. This does not mean that they have the same nutritional properties as pasta, bread, grains, and rice. These foods are also carbohydrates, but have a different effect on the body due to processing that strips out the dietary fiber and nutrients. What is left is a starchy food that spikes blood sugar levels and lacks any sort of nutritional punch.

Eat carbohydrates. Just make sure they are in the form of whole fruits, vegetables, and minimally processed grains. Choose foods that are high in fiber (4-5 grams per serving), have not been significantly altered from their natural state, and consume them in appropriate portions (enough to fill one cupped hand).

Eat fat. Fat is not the enemy. Unhealthy fat is what causes negative effects in the body. Fats occurring naturally in plants and animals are healthy in appropriate portions (healthy = meat from grass-fed or pasture-raised animals and fatty fruit like avocado; portions should be about the size of the palm).

Avoid fatty foods that are highly processed; they often have added fat or fat made in a lab.

Protein is the building block of muscle, bones, cartilage, skin and blood. Protein is also used by the body to make hormones and and other body chemicals. It comes from a variety of sources. Consume protein from a variety of sources, including meat, poultry, seafood, beans, eggs, nuts and seeds.

"Eat more fruits and vegetables."

PROTEIN

Protein is one of the three macro nutrients, along with carbohydrates and fats. There are many debates about how much protein a person should consume, how often it should be eaten, when is the best time to have protein, and what is the best food source for protein. The information regarding protein is often confusing and contradictory.

Mighty Oak Athletic does not promote the a one-solution-fits-all approach to health. While humans have many general physical characteristics in common, there is also a large amount of nuance and variety in each individual's body composition. Body chemistry is simply not that simple!

To answer the question of protein consumption, it is important too start with the end in mind. What is the intended outcome? Is the goal weight loss? Add muscle mass? Perform in a professional sport? Increase longevity? Improve health span?

The goal must be defined before asking the question. Once a target has been set, it becomes easier to develop a nutritional plan that incorporates the proper amount of protein, with the correct frequency, at the right time, and from the best source.

This may seem like a non-answer. It is a push to prompt readers to begin asking better questions. *How much protein should I eat?* is a poor question. *How much protein should I consume everyday if I plan to dance at my great-granddaughter's wedding 60 years from now?* is a more easily answered question.

Define the goal.

> *"Once a target has been set, it becomes easier to develop a nutritional plan that incorporates the proper amount of protein, with the correct frequency, at the right time, and from the best source."*

Meat

Vegetarian. Pescatarian. Flexatarian. There are a lot of approaches to eating that shun meat in the diet. Some people do not meat for religious or ethical reasons. These are all completely reasonable reasons to not consume meat. Other people, however, avoid meat because of the perceived health detriments of consuming meat. This is both right and wrong.

Unhealthy animals produce unhealthy meat. Healthy animals have meat that is loaded with healthy fats, essential proteins, vitamins and minerals.

It is important to source meat that comes from animals raised on a diet that is natural to their species - cows are built to eat grass, not grain. When animals like cows are force-fed grain, it causes all sorts of physical problems for the animal. Subsequently, the cow is then loaded up with antibiotics and other medications to keep it "healthy." These drugs make their way into the animals' meat, and onto consumers' plates. There is a saying: It's not what you eat; it's what you eat ate. Eat healthy animals.

Some animals, cattle specifically, are often given growth hormones to expedite the amount of time it takes to get from calf to slaughter weight. Again, these drugs make their way into the animal's meat and onto consumers' plates. Those drug-infused foods wreak havoc on the human body.

Eat a variety of meat - different animals, different cuts, and various organs. Not all meat has the same nutritional profile. A serving (about the size of the palm) of lean cut of beef can have 25 grams of protein, 10 grams of healthy fat, and is loaded with iron and zinc. Pork is often high in vitamin B1 which is great for the nervous system and the brain. Lamb is rich in vitamin B12 which helps make red blood cells and keeps nerve cells healthy. Beef liver is rich in vitamins C and B6.

"Healthy animals have meat that is loaded with healthy fats, essential proteins, vitamins and minerals."

Poultry

Chickens were one of the first animals that humans domesticated. They are fairly easy to manage and are prolific egg layers. Chickens are also meaty birds that provide copious amounts of lean protein.

Eat light meat (chicken breast) and dark meat (chicken leg and thigh) to get the benefit of different nutritional offerings from chicken.

Need more protein and less fat? A serving of chicken breast meat has approximately 30 grams of protein and 3 grams of fat. It is also loaded with vitamin B3 for healthy skin and vitamin B6 for improved immune function.

Want to feel full longer from a fattier cut of poultry? A serving of chicken thigh has 25 grams of protein and 10 grams of fat. The dark meat has the nutrient taurine which lowers inflammation, and vitamins A and K for bone health.

"Eat light meat and dark meat to get the benefit of different nutritional offerings from chicken."

Seafood

Fresh seafood has become increasingly more available to people living away from the coast or other bodies of water. This is partly due to the increase in farm-raised fish. While farm-raised fish has made it possible to provide more lower-cost food available to a larger number of people, it has also decreased the nutritional profile of a lot of the seafood that people consume.

Opt for wild caught seafood whenever possible. Wild caught seafood eats a diet natural to their species and is subsequently healthier than fish that are fed man-made food and the antibiotics the fish often need to keep from getting sick on an unnatural food source.

Just like meat and poultry, eat a variety of seafood to get a full spectrum of protein, fat, vitamins and minerals.

A serving of wild caught salmon is loaded with protein (40 grams), healthy fats (omega-3), B vitamins, vitamin C, potassium (regulates fluid balance), and magnesium (improves brain function and mood).

Lake Superior whitefish is a great source of phosphorus (strong bones and teeth) and zinc (healing of wounds).

Lobster is loaded with copper (forms collagen) and selenium (powerful antioxidant).

> *"Wild caught seafood eats a diet natural to their species and is subsequently healthier than fish that are fed man-made food and the antibiotics the fish often need to keep from getting sick on their unnatural food source."*

Beans

Beans are affectionately referred to as the magical fruit. And not just because it rhymes with toot! Beans are high in protein, fiber, and a myriad of vitamins and minerals. Variety is again the key to unlocking the nutritional benefits that beans have to offer.

Chickpeas, a.k.a. Garbanzo beans, are high in vitamin B9 (production of DNA and RNA), manganese (bone health), and iron (carries oxygen to muscles).

Eat black beans for magnesium (energy production).

Peanuts - yes, they are a legume - have high levels of vitamin E (antioxidant).

"Beans are high in protein, fiber, and a myriad of vitamins and minerals."

Eggs

Eggs are often wrongly perceived as an unhealthy food. The enemy is said to be the yolk, which has the fat and cholesterol. The opposite is true! The yolk is home to the healthiest parts of the egg.

A whole egg provides 6 grams of protein, 5 grams of healthy fat, cholesterol (builds cell membranes and stimulates hormone production in the body), and vitamin D (calcium absorption).

*A note on cholesterol: It is now believed that dietary cholesterol has a minimal effect on blood cholesterol levels in most people. There is compelling research from numerous sources that show genetic make up is what drives blood cholesterol levels, not food. Eat the yolk!

"Eat the yolk!"

Soy

Soybeans are a good source of protein, fiber, fat, vitamins and minerals. Soy comes in a variety of forms - soybeans, tofu, tempeh, edamame, yogurt, and milk. These different forms have varying nutritional profiles.

A serving of tempeh has 20 grams of protein and high levels of vitamin B2 (cell growth). Edamame is a great source of vitamin B9 (crucial during early pregnancy).

Soy is a hot topic in health and nutrition circles. There are many people (Mighty Oak included) that have concerns about the overconsumption of soy. Do some research and make an educated decision about including soy as part of a balanced diet. People getting protein from soy should consider consuming it in small portions a few times a week.

"People getting protein from soy should consider consuming it in small portions a few times a week."

Nuts

Nuts are another food source that have gotten a bad rap lately. This stems from the increase in incidences of allergic reactions to tree nuts in recent years. The reason for this increase is still being studied and the results are inconclusive.

This is unfortunate, because nuts are safe for most people to consume. Nuts are some of the most nutritious foods on the planet! They are a good source of protein, fat, fiber, vitamins and minerals. Like most protein sources, variety offers an array of different nutritional benefits.

A serving of almonds delivers a healthy balance of protein (6 grams), fat (14 grams), carbohydrates (6 grams), and fiber (4 grams). They are also loaded with vitamin E (protects cells against free radicals - unstable atoms that can damage cells and cause the body to age and get sick).

Walnuts are a great source of alpha-linolenic acid (ALA) which is an essential omega-3 fatty acid that is important for heart health.

Cashews are high in magnesium (brain function) and have been found to improve blood pressure.

"Nuts are some of the most nutritious foods on the planet!"

Seeds

Eat seeds for a plant-based boost of protein, fiber, fat, and minerals like: phosphorus, calcium, magnesium, and iron. Eat a variety of seeds - sunflower, pumpkin, chia, sesame, hemp, chia.

A handful of mixed of sunflower and pumpkin seeds make a great snack to stave off hunger pangs and give the body a boost of satiating fat and energy producing protein.

Mix chia seeds or ground flaxseed into oatmeal and smoothies to add protein without adding a large number of calories or volume to the meal.

Sprinkle sesame seeds onto salads and stir fry's for a boost of iron (growth of red blood cells).

"Eat a variety of seeds - sunflower, pumpkin, chia, sesame, hemp, chia."

Strength

Be strong to be useful. It requires lean muscle mass to be strong. Protein is the fuel that builds muscles mass. Eat protein to build muscle, get strong, and be useful.

Consume protein from both animal and plant-based food, as well from a variety of types of food. Mix it up to provide the body with a full spectrum of protein, fat, fiber, vitamins and minerals.

Eat protein to build muscle, get strong, and be useful."

FAT

Fat - the good, the bad, and the ugly. Fat is terrible to eat! Fat is extremely healthy to eat! Wait. What?

The story on fat has changed over the years. In the 1990's, fat was vilified and said to cause every health-related ailment known to man. In the 2000's, fat was celebrated and suggested that it be consumed at every meal. The experts even said fat should be liberally applied to the skin, hair, and nails!

The truth lies somewhere in the middle. Fat is not good or bad. Some types of dietary fat can be very healthy when consumed as part of a balanced diet. Others are extremely hazardous to human health and should be avoided. Let's take a look at the three types of dietary fat.

The Good - Unsaturated Fat

Unsaturated fat is easily recognized; it is in a liquid form - think olive oil. Unsaturated fat can improve cholesterol levels, lower inflammation, and has many other healthy benefits. Unsaturated fats are mainly found in foods from plants, like nuts, seeds, and vegetable oils.

There are two types of unsaturated fat - mono and poly. Monounsaturated fat can be found in olives, almonds, avocados, and pumpkin seeds. Polyunsaturated fat is consumed by eating sunflower seeds, walnuts, and fish.

The Bad - Saturated Fat

Saturated fat is solid at room temperature - think butter. Some level of saturated fat is found in most foods - chicken has a little and beef has a lot. Saturated fats are mainly found in red meat, dairy products, and some oils like coconut and palm oil. Saturated fat can be part of a healthy diet if it is consumed in moderation by eating meat from grass-fed and free-range animals. Too many people have diets heavy in factory raised meat, as well as diets with large amounts of butter and cheese from unhealthy cows.

The Ugly - Trans Fat

Trans fats can occur naturally in animals. This is not what is dangerous to human health. Industrial fats processed to make liquid fat more solid is nasty stuff.

This is done by adding hydrogen. Be on the lookout for partially hydrogenated oil. Many restaurants fry food in these oils. Trans fat oils give food an improved taste and texture, but at a heavy cost. Eating trans fat will significantly increase the chances for heart disease, stroke, and type 2 diabetes.

So, is it healthy or unhealthy to eat foods high in fat? It depends. Food that can be traced back to flora and fauna is generally full of healthy fats and nutrients.

Always be able to answer the questions: "What is it?" and "Where does it come from?" Yes, it is a Dorito that comes from

Walmart. And it is delicious! But can it be traced back to a natural source or does it go through processing in a factory or lab? Food that comes from a factory or a lab is best avoided. Focus on consuming fats - not too much - that come mostly from plants and healthy animals.

> *"Focus on consuming fats - not too much - that come mostly from plants and healthy animals."*

Conditioning

Conditioning is physical training that makes it possible for the body's systems and organs to perform at their optimal level. It is often high intensity interval training like the Tabata Protocol, or slower distance training like jogging and swimming.

Conditioning training challenges and improves the body's cardiovascular, immune, nervous, endocrine, digestive and respiratory systems, as well as muscular endurance and bone strength. This type of training requires proper nutrition to fuel the activities.

The optimal fuel is a mix of carbohydrates and fat. Think of carbohydrates as the quick burning kindling that will ignite the training fire. Fat is the big logs burned to sustain the training fire for longer periods of time.

It is important to have a diet that includes a balance of complex carbohydrates and unsaturated fats. Too many carbs and too few fats will enable the body to train for intense bursts over a short period of time, but will not provide the body the fuel it needs to perform for an extended period of time. Too many fats and not enough carbs will make it challenging for the body to jumpstart training.

The optimal balance will have the right amount of carbohydrates to fuel the start of a training, and then allowing the body to switch to burning fat to fuel the remainder of the session.

The optimal ratio of carbohydrates to fat will vary for each person. Experiment with eating more of one and less of another leading up to a training session. Make notes on how the body feels and responds to the training. While there are other factors like sleep, recovery between sessions, stress, type of training, etc. that can effect the body, a simple food journal will often uncover the ideal combination of carbs and fats that work best for each person.

"Conditioning is physical training that makes it possible for the body's systems and organs to perform at their optimal level."

CARBOHYDRATE

Carbohydrates can be the most confusing piece in the nutrition puzzle. This is primarily because carbohydrates are found in both healthy and unhealthy foods. While there has been a lot of talk about low-carb and no-carb diets, carbohydrates are absolutely part of a balanced and healthy diet.

Carbohydrates provide the body with glucose, which is converted to energy used to support the body's functions and physical activity. That being said, most Americans eat significantly too many carbohydrates. Americans consume in excess of 130 pounds of grains a year! The standard American diet is comprised of carbohydrates that are highly-processed and refined (bran and germ removed). These carbs are usually consumed in the form of white bread, flour tortillas, pasta, white rice, and sugary cereals.

Refined carbohydrates cause a significant spike in blood sugar and insulin. Over-consumption of refined carbohydrates can lead to an increased risk for heart disease, Type 2 diabetes, digestive problems, and obesity.

The better option is to opt for whole grain foods (bran, germ, and endosperm intact). Whole grains are higher in fiber and slower to effect blood sugar and insulin levels.

Focus not only on the quantity of carbs consumed, but also on the quality. The key is to eat the right foods and to consume carbs from a high-quality food source. The best sources include fruits and vegetables, whole grains, and beans. High quality carbohydrates provide dietary fiber, as well as an essential vitamins and minerals.

What do high-quality carbohydrates look like?

- Whole, organic fruits and vegetables - avoid juices! It is not a good habit to drink sugar. Juices often strip away the fiber. Fiber allows for slower digestion and subsequently a lower spike in blood sugar.
- Old fashioned oatmeal (avoid instant!) and steel cut oats. Read the nutrition label and aim for 4-5 grams of fiber per serving, and no added sugar.
- Go easy on the bread. Even whole wheat bread is highly processed, and store bought options can be loaded with salt and sugar.
- Consume rice with at least 3 grams of fiber. This generally includes wild and brown rice options.
- Experiment with more complex grains. Try farro, barley, amaranth, millet, kaput, spelt, sorghum, teff, freekeh, quinoa, bulger, rye, or fonio.
- Add beans to the grains. Pairing grains with beans helps the body metabolize the carbs better. The proteins in rice and beans combine to make a complete protein, which supplies all the necessary amino acids (building blocks of protein).
- Go easy on the potatoes. Potatoes are nutritious, but most Americans consume far too many at one meal, as well as far too many each week. And French fries are not nutritious!
- Avoid store bought products. Make bread, pasta, cookies, and grains from scratch as often as possible; this will

control the quality of the ingredients and improve the overall quality of the food.

"Carbohydrates can be the most confusing piece in the nutrition puzzle."

Vegetable

A vegetable is a plant, or part of a plant, that is edible. In general, if it has seeds, it is a fruit. Squash, tomatoes, and avocado are examples of foods that are commonly considered vegetables, but are technically fruits. Peppers are berries and mushrooms are fungus!

Make vegetables the main part of any meal or snack. A serving size of vegetables is the amount that will fit into two hands cupped together.

It is important to eat a large quantity of vegetables, and also a large variety of vegetables. Think of eating the rainbow. Have a different color vegetable each meal.

Try artichokes, arugula, asparagus, book chop, broccoli, cabbage, cauliflower, chives, fennel, leeks, okra, parsnips, radicchio, radishes, watercress, and yams. Opt for organic vegetables whenever possible, especially spinach, kale, and celery which are all heavily sprayed with pesticides.

"A serving size of vegetables is the amount that will fit into two cupped hands together."

Fruit

A fruit is the sweet and fleshy part of a plant that is edible. Fruits have seeds. Avocados, squash, and tomatoes all fruits.

Fruits are often high in sugar, but the spike in blood sugar is often blunted by the fiber that is in the fruit. This is why it is preferable to eat whole fruit and to avoid juices. Don't drink sugar! A serving size of fruit is the amount that will fit into one cupped hand.

Fruit is loaded with vitamins and minerals, but needs to be eaten in moderation due to the higher levels of sugar. It is also preferable to consume fruit earlier in the day to allow the body time to burn the sugars as fuel during daily activity.

Like vegetables, eat the fruit rainbow. Have different color fruits throughout the day. Try apricot, blackberry, cherry, grape, huckleberry, kiwi, lychee, mandarin, mango, musk melon, papaya, plantain, quince, ugli fruit, and yuzu. Opt for organic fruit whenever possible, especially strawberries, nectarines, apples, grapes, cherries, peaches, pears, peppers, and tomatoes which are all heavily sprayed with pesticides.

"A serving size of fruit is the amount that will fit into one cupped hand."

Grain

Grains are the edible seeds from grasses and plants. Common grains are wheat, oats, corn, rice and barley. Less common grains include tiff, barley, sorghum, rye, millet, triticale, amaranth, buckwheat, quinoa.

Grains are part of a healthy and balanced diet. The challenge is that most Americans eat significantly too many carbohydrates. Americans consume in excess of 130 pounds of grains a year! A serving size of grains is the amount that will fit into one cupped hand.

The standard American diet is comprised of carbohydrates that are highly-processed and refined (bran and germ removed). These carbs are usually consumed in the form of white bread, flour tortillas, pasta, white rice, and sugary cereals.

Refined carbohydrates cause a significant spike in blood sugar and insulin. Over-consumption of refined carbohydrates can lead to an increased risk for heart disease, Type 2 diabetes, digestive problems, and obesity.

The better option is to choose whole grain foods (bran, germ, and endosperm intact). Whole grains are higher in fiber and slower to effect blood sugar and insulin levels.

Old fashioned oatmeal and steel cut oats are an example of whole grains. Avoid instant oatmeal! Read the nutrition label and aim for 4-5 grams of fiber per serving and no added sugar.

Go easy on the bread. Even whole wheat bread is highly processed, and store bought options can be loaded with salt and sugar.

Consume rice with at least 3 grams of fiber. This generally includes wild and brown rice options.

Experiment with more complex grains. Try farro, barley, amaranth, millet, kaput, spelt, sorghum, teff, freekeh, quinoa, bulger, rye, or fonio.

Add beans to the grains. Pairing grains with beans helps the body metabolize the carbs better. The proteins in rice and beans combine to make a complete protein, which supplies all the necessary amino acids (building blocks of protein).

"A serving size of grains is the amount that will fit into one cupped hand."

Health

What is a reasonable definition of health? Health is all of the body's organs playing nice together. What it takes to achieve that optimal interplay is complex and can vary for each person. There are some basic principals, however, that can be applied by most people most of the time.

1. Eat more fruits and vegetables. Most people either eat too few fruits and vegetables, or not enough variety. Add a serving of a new fruit or vegetable to each meal and health will improve. Select organic whenever possible.

2. Eat less grains. Most people eat far too many grains, especially highly processed and refined grains. Aim for one serving of whole grains per day. Add in a variety of grains. Break out of the basic wheat, rice, and corn. Eat whole grains whenever possible.

3. Eat more fat from plants, nuts, and seeds. Drizzle olive oil onto vegetables or snack on roasted pecans and pumpkin seeds.

4. Eat more protein. Consume protein from a variety of sources like meat, poultry, seafood, eggs, nuts, seeds, and beans. Eat grass-fed, organic, and wild caught options whenever possible.

5. Drink more water. Urine should be the color of lemonade - light yellow.

6. Avoid alcohol. Alcohol has very few health benefits and lots of health negatives.

7. Move more throughout the day. Take walks in the morning, afternoon and evening. Do some strenuous conditioning activity a few times a week. Lift something heavy a couple of times per week. Stretch and work on mobility most days.

8. Sleep consistently. Go to bed at the same time every night. Shut down electronics one hour before bed. Have a pre-sleep routine to calm the mind and prepare for rest.

"Health is all of the body's organs playing nice together."

VITAMINS

Vitamins are organic compounds that humans need for the body to grow and function properly. They are needed in small amounts consistently each day. Most vitamins come from food and are best consumed through diet, not supplements. Getting vitamins from food sources makes them more effective.

"Vitamins are organic compounds that humans need for the body to grow and function properly."

Vitamin A

Keeps eyes healthy, boosts immune system, reduces aches, and builds strong bones.

Food Sources of Vitamin A

Eggs, kale, spinach, broccoli, and orange colored fruits and vegetables like carrot, sweet potato, squash, mango, papaya.

Vitamin B1 (thiamine)

Boosts energy, fights depression, improves concentration and memory.

Food Sources of Vitamin B1
Trout, pork chops, black beans, acorn squash.

Vitamin B2 (riboflavin)

Breaks down fat, protein, and carbohydrates into energy; maintains healthy hair, skin, and nails.

Food Sources of Vitamin B2
Beef liver, chicken breast, salmon, eggs.

Vitamin B3 (niacin)

Improves cholesterol, lowers triglycerides, improves skin function.

Food Sources of Vitamin B3
Beef liver, chicken breast, tuna, salmon, anchovies.

Vitamin B5 (pantothenic acid)

Improves function of nervous system, aids the production of red blood cells, contributes to a healthy digestive tract.

Food Sources of Vitamin B5
Chicken liver, lobster, lentils, eggs

Vitamin B6 (pyridoxine)

Improves immune system, circulation, and mood.

Food Sources of Vitamin B6
Ricotta cheese, chicken liver, tuna, carrots, spinach.

Vitamin B7 (biotin)

Breaks down fat, protein, and carbohydrates into energy; maintains healthy hair, skin, and nails.

Food Sources of Vitamin B7
Walnuts, peanuts, eggs, beef liver, avocado, salmon.

Vitamin B9 (folic acid)

Aids in the production of red blood cells, assists in the formation of RNA and DNA

Foods Sources of Vitamin B9
Spinach, Brussels sprouts, broccoli, peanuts, beef liver, eggs.

Vitamin B12 (cobalamin)

Aids in development of brain and nerve cells, assists in the production of red blood cells.

Food Sources of Vitamin B12
Trout, salmon, eggs.

Vitamin C

Boosts immune system, growth and repair of body tissue, lowers blood pressure.

Food Sources of Vitamin C
Bell pepper, cantaloupe, kiwi, tomato, broccoli, Brussels sprouts, lemon, orange.

Vitamin D

Aids in calcium absorption to improve bone health, reduces inflammation.

Food Sources of Vitamin D
Sunshine, sardines, salmon, eggs

Vitamin E

Powerful antioxidant, boosts immunity, builds healthy skin and eyes

Food sources of Vitamin E
Almonds, peanuts, sunflower seeds, spinach, broccoli.

Vitamin K

Helps the blood to clot, aids in calcium metabolism, supports bone strength

Food Sources of Vitamin K
Kale, parsley, cabbage, broccoli, Brussels sprouts.

Choline

Forms cell membranes, aids communication between neurons.

Food Sources of Choline
Beef liver, cauliflower, broccoli, eggs.

"Most vitamins come from food and are best consumed through diet, not supplement."

MINERALS

Minerals are the elements that humans need for the body to grow and function properly. They are needed in small amounts consistently each day. Most minerals come from food and are best consumed through diet, not supplements. Getting minerals from food sources makes them more effective.

"Minerals are elements that humans need for the body to grow and function properly."

Calcium

Builds and maintains strong bones.

Food Sources of Calcium
Kale, okra, cheese, yogurt

Chloride

Maintain balance of body fluids, aids in stomach digestion.

Food Sources of Chloride
Sea salt, tomatoes, celery, olives, seaweed

Chromium

Enhances protein, carbohydrate, and fat metabolism; improves insulin sensitivity

Food Sources of Chromium
Mussels, broccoli, beef, Brazil nuts

Copper

Aids in development of red blood cells, builds healthy blood vessels, supports healthy nerves.

Food Sources of Copper
Beef liver, oysters, Shiitake mushrooms, lobster, kale

Fluoride

Strengthens tooth enamel, prevents growth of oral bacteria.

Food Sources of Fluoride
Black tea, coffee, shrimp, raisins, cooked oatmeal.

Iodine

Maintain proper thyroid function.

Food Sources of Iodine
Cod, tuna, shrimp, seaweed, iodized salt

Iron

Aids in development of hemoglobin and myoglobin for red blood cells.

Food Sources of Iron
Dark meat poultry, beef, oysters.

Magnesium

Aids in enzyme reactions, regulates blood pressure, supports immune system

Food Sources of Magnesium
Halibut, spinach, potatoes, almonds, cashews.

Manganese

Helps form connective tissue, helps form sex hormones.

Food Sources of Manganese
Mussels, brown rice, chickpeas, hazelnuts, spinach, pineapple, potatoes.

Molybdenum

Helps break down toxic substances in the body.

Food Sources of Molybdenum
Black eye peas, lima beans, potatoes, bananas.

Phosphorus

Aids in formation of strong bones and teeth.

Food Sources of Phosphorus
Turkey, sardines, pumpkin seeds, sunflower seeds, Brazil nuts, quinoa, lentils.

Potassium

Helps regulate fluid balance and water retention

Food Sources of Potassium
Cooked spinach, cooked, broccoli, bananas, potatoes, sweet potatoes, mushrooms, peas, cucumbers.

Selenium

Helps protect the thyroid from oxidative damage.

Food sources of Selenium
Brazil nuts, ham, turkey, eggs, brown rice, sunflower seeds.

Sodium

Aids in conduction of nerve impulses, helps contract and relax muscles.

Food Sources of Sodium
Sea salt.

Sulfur

Aids in making and repair of DNA, improves skin and reduces acne.

Food Sources of Sulfur
Duck, scallops, kidney beans, walnuts, cheddar cheese, oats, coconut milk, ginger root.

Zinc

Boosts immunity, aids in wound repair, stimulates cell growth.

Food Sources of Zinc
Oysters, crab, pork tenderloin, baked beans, pumpkin seeds, cashews

"Most minerals come from food and are best consumed through diet, not supplements."

ONE MONTH TO IMPROVED HEALTH

Month one is all about the reset. It is an opportunity to reprogram the mind and recondition the body. It will be challenging. It is supposed to be challenging. Challenging is what makes it great! If it was not challenging, everyone would do it. Then it would not be special. Lean into the hard. Make the change and come out a healthier and happier person in 30 days.

Nutrition

What is the one lesson to take away from this book? Eat more fruits and vegetables. That's it! Adding more fresh fruits and vegetables to the plate will improve nutrition by adding essential vitamins and minerals to the diet, and by decreasing the amount of non-healthy foods consumed. This one improvement has double the return on investment!

Movement

What does healthy human movement look like? A body that can move with mobility, agility, balance, coordination, strength, and endurance. There needs to be a full range of movement at the joints, an ability to move proficiently on land *and* water, able to balance on a variety of uneven surfaces, lift heavy objects without getting injured, play sports and games, defend itself, and perform the basic human movements required for activity in everyday life - squat down, push up, pull up, lift an object off the ground, and carry an object for distance.

Recovery

Rest and recovery are the unsung heroes in the Circles of Life. Make rejuvenation a priority. The time spent training breaks down the body. During rest is when the body can repair and grow stronger. Give the body ample time to rebuild and recover. Take time to rest!

Final thought

Stick to the plan. Be patient. Be consistent. And get some rest!

MIGHTY OAK ATHLETIC

Training Program - Month 1

MOBILITY	Around the Clock			
	1 set of 12 repetitions			
CORE	Bird Dog	Shoulder Tap	Scissor	Cross Punch
	1 set of 10 repetitions per side			
CONDITIONING	Knee-to-Elbow	Toe-Squat-Sky	Jacob Ladder	Twist Press
	1 set of 10 repetitions per side			
POWER	Squat Jump	Sumo Jump	Lunge Jump	Side Jump
	1 set of 10 repetitions			
STRENGTH	Squat	Push Up	Toe Touch	Row
WEEK 1	*5x10*	*5x10*	*5x10*	*5x10*
WEEK 2	*4x12*	*4x12*	*4x12*	*4x12*
WEEK 3	*3x15*	*3x15*	*3x15*	*3x15*
WEEK 4	*2x25*	*2x25*	*2x25*	*2x25*

MONTH 1 TRAINING PROGRAM

The Month 1 Training Program has mobility training one day a week, and strength and conditioning training twice a week. The mobility training session can be completed in 10 minutes. The strength and condition training can be completed in 20 minutes.

On the other four non-training days, make time to walk, bike, swim, play sports, or participate in any other activities that are fun and fatiguing. Break a sweat, laugh, and enjoy moving.

All of the movement videos can be found online at: https://www.mightyoakathletic.com/exercises

Have questions? Join the Mighty Oak Athletic Facebook group for help with FAQs and motivation: https://www.facebook.com/pg/MightyOakAthletic/groups

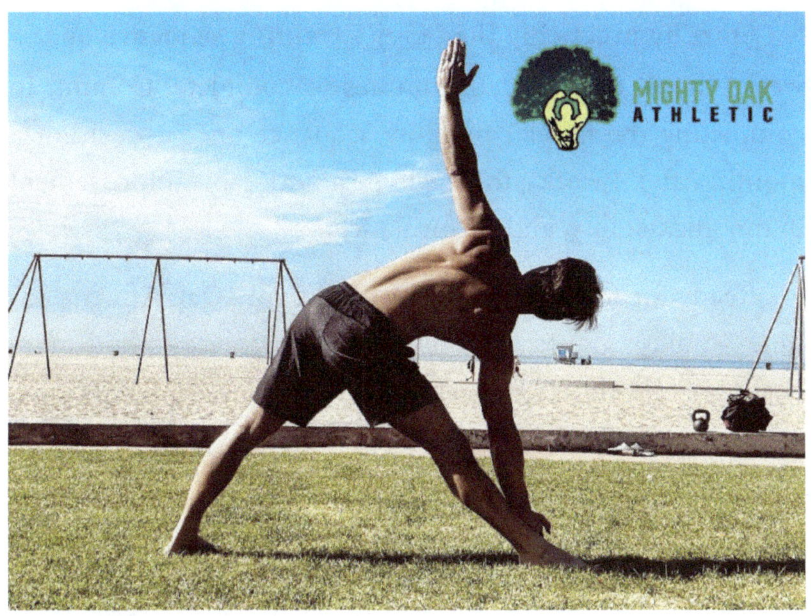

MOBILITY TRAINING

Mobility is a must. Remember the formula: *Good Mobility = Good Movement Patterns = Less Injury = Ability to Move = Good Health*

Mobility improves movement patterns and range of motion. This will improve performance and decrease injuries. Not only should mobility work be included as part of a warm up, it also needs to be given a dedicated day in a training schedule.

Mighty Oak Athletic provides numerous mobility training videos on MightyOakAthletic.com and the Mighty Oak Athletic Vimeo and YouTube pages.

Start by practicing the <u>Level 1</u> training sequence once a week. It will only take 10 minutes to complete. Commit to completing the Level 1 mobility sequence once a week for a month. After 4 weeks, there will be a noticeable improvement in mobility, agility, and performance.

Ready for more mobility? Great! Mighty Oak Athletic has nine <u>mobility videos available for FREE</u> online to add more challenge and variety to the training.

STRENGTH AND CONDITIONING TRAINING

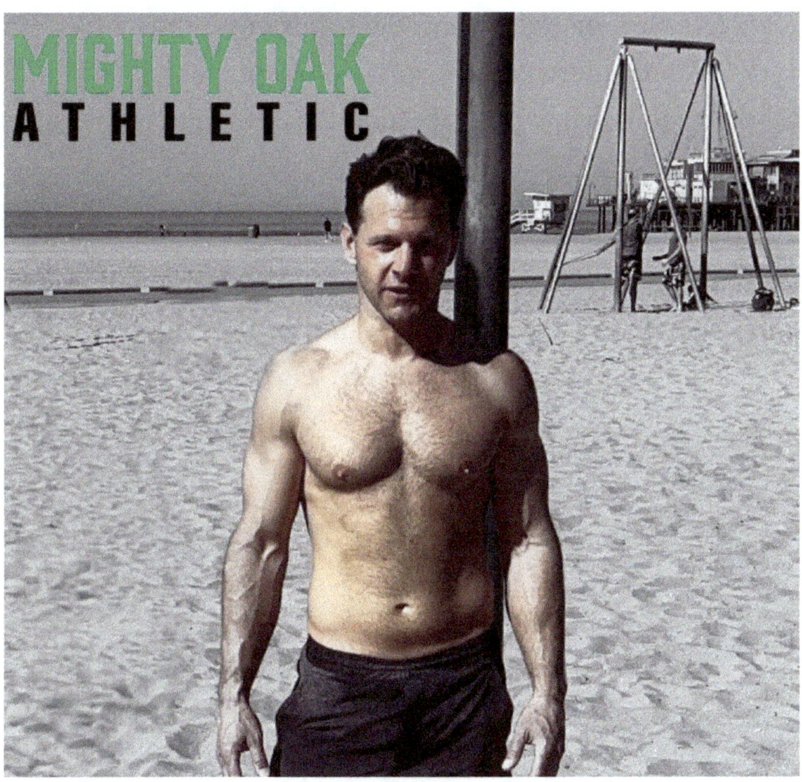

Strength training is generally associated with lifting weights. This is a very narrow view of building strength, and leaves little latitude in designing a well-rounded strength training program as part of a healthy movement program.

Another challenge is that strength training is linked to how much weight a person can move. Increasing measurable strength does not necessarily correlate to improved movement or physical health.

It is useful to reframe strength training as *training for functional strength* - strength that can be applied to daily performance. As an example, using the leg extension machine in a gym will build muscular strength and size in the leg. It will not, however, do much to improve functional strength in the legs.

Functional strength requires a symphony of balance, coordination, and reciprocal muscles working in concert to move the body in an efficient and effective manner. Humans do not jump by simply flexing the knee; they use the hip, knee, and ankle joints to load the legs and spring upward.

MOBILITY

Movement starts with mobility - the body's ability to move freely and easily.

Without a healthy, full range of motion, the body cannot function at it's best. Limited mobility leads to a limited range of motion. When the motions of the body are restricted, injuries occur as the body compensates and moves in inefficient ways. When the body is injured, overall movement will decrease. Lack of movement leads to a decline in health.

Around the Clock

The Around the Clock is a great movement to warm up the shoulder, hip, knee, and ankle joints. Start standing with feet hip-width distance apart. Pivot on the balls of the feet, turn the hips to the right, and reach up with both hands towards an imaginary 1:00. Twist back to the starting position. Repeat reaching towards 2:00, returning to the starting position, reaching towards 3:00, etc. until touching all 12 points on the clock. Complete one set of 12 repetitions.

CORE

The core is the center of the body, approximately from the hip to the sternum, all the way around the abdomen. Many movements start at the core and work outward towards the extremities. It is important to build a strong core, not just the six pack abs, but also the smaller stabilizing muscles found deep in the belly. These under-appreciated muscles keep the body moving strong and pain-free.

When strengthening the muscles around the core, make sure to work all sides of the midsection. This includes the muscles that run from the sternum to the pelvis; along the sides from the ribs to the hip; and across the lower back.

<u>Bird Dog</u>

The Bird Dog strengthens the muscles across the lower back. Start with hands and knees on the ground, forming a table top with the back. While maintaining a flat back, and keeping hips and shoulders parallel to the ground, simultaneously lift the right arm and left leg up. Imagine pressing the foot into the back wall and the hand into the front wall. Simultaneously lower both the arm and leg down, returning to table top position. Repeat with the left arm and the right leg. Complete one set of 10 repetitions per side; 20 total repetitions.

Shoulder Tap

Shoulder taps build the stabilizer muscles along the front of the abdomen, the deep supporting muscles around what is commonly referred to as the six pack. Focus on keeping the hips and shoulders parallel to the floor throughout the movement. Avoid twist and rocking from side-to-side.

Start with the hands and feet on the floor in a push up position. Take a moment to check the alignment of the body. The shoulders should be down and away from the ears; the shoulder, elbow, and wrist should be in a straight line; the tailbone tucked and the muscles around the bellybutton feel switched on; the kneecaps are zipped up to engage the muscles in the thigh; the heel is directly over the ball of the foot.

While maintaining hips and shoulders parallel to the ground, lift the right hand from the ground and tap the left shoulder. Place the right hand back down under control. Repeat with the left hand and opposite shoulder. Complete one set of 10 repetitions per side.

Scissors

Scissors, also known as flutter kicks, strengthen the muscles in the hips and lower abdomen. Move the legs in a smooth and controlled manner. Keep the tempo methodical and avoid moving too quickly and straining the small muscles in the hips.

Start in a seated position. Lean back to the elbows and place the legs out straight. Lift the feet up six inches off of the ground. Begin kicking the feet in an alternating manner, as if flutter kicking in water. Keep the toes pointed and the rhythm consistent. Complete one set of 10 repetitions per side.

<u>Cross Punch</u>

Twisting movements improve mobility in the spine, as well as strengthen the muscles along the side of the abdomen. Start the motion at the shoulders and turn the chest to the side while keeping the rest of the body facing forward.

Begin in a seated position with knees bent and the feet flat on the floor. Turn the shoulders to the right and reach the left hand across the body, punching to the right. Twist back to the center. Repeat on the opposite side by turning the shoulders to the left and reaching the right hand across the body, punching to the left. Twist back to the center. Complete one set of 10 repetitions per side.

CONDITIONING

Conditioning is the use of large muscle groups in a coordinated way that raises the heart rate and respiration while increasing the flow of oxygen and blood throughout the body. Confusing? Complete 25 jumping jacks. That sensation after doing the jumping jacks is the body's response to cardiovascular conditioning.

Conditioning training (often referred to as cardio training) is a great way to strengthen the heart, improve lung capacity, boost energy, improve mood, strengthen the immune system, and leads to better sleep.

Knee-to-Elbow

The Knee-to-Elbow is a spinal rotation movement that strengthens the hips, loosens up the sine, and improves range of lotion in the upper back. It also challenges balance by working on one foot, as well as coordination by using opposite sides of the body.

Begin standing with feet hip width distance apart. Lift the elbows high out in front of the chest. Twist the center of the chest to the left while simultaneously raising the left knee in the direction of the right elbow. Lower the leg and repeat by turning to the right and bringing up the right leg to meet the left elbow. Complete one set of 10 repetitions per side.

Toe-Squat-Sky

This is a total body movement the strengthens the hips, rump, legs, and shoulders. It moves the body through all of the primary motions - hinge, squat, push, and pull.

Start with the feet just slightly wider than hip width apart. Press the rump back, hingeing at the waist, to reach down and touch the toes. Bring the hips forward and return to standing tall. Next, sit down into a squat by bringing the elbows between the knees. Return to standing tall and press the hands overhead while coming up. That is one repetition. Complete one set of 10 repetitions.

Jacobs Ladder

The Jacobs Ladder is a great movement to improve balance and coordination, as well as drive the heart rate up and get the lungs heaving. It will also strengthen the hip muscles and improve mobility in the shoulders.

Start in a standing position with feet hip width distance apart. Lift the left knee to hip height while simultaneously pressing the right hand straight up overhead. As if climbing a ladder or running in place, alternate lifting opposite hands and knees. Complete one set of 10 repetitions per side.

Twist Press

The Twist Press builds strength in the shoulders, core, and hips. It also improves mobility in the back and loosens the spine. It is important to turn the entire torso from side-to-side, as well as making sure to pivot on the balls of the feet. Start the motion by swiveling the hips and allowing the rest of the body to follow.

Start in a standing position with feet hip width distance apart. Bring the hands in front of the chest. Turn the hips to the left, pivoting on the balls of the feet, and pressing the hands up at a 45 degree angle. Twist back through the center and immediately turn to the right, repeating the motion on the other side. Complete one set of 10 repetitions per side.

POWER

Power = Strength x Speed. This style of training requires explosive movements. It is not about lifting a maximal amount of weight. Power training is about moving the heaviest weight possible at a maximum speed. Often times, using bodyweight movements will be challenging enough to develop power. Olympic lifts like the clean or the snatch are examples of weighted power movements. These movements are highly technical and require proper coaching to execute the movements safely and effectively. Start out with bodyweight movements to build explosive power while keeping the risk for injury to a minimum.

<u>Squat Jump</u>

The Squat Jump is a movement that is easy to master and will have a huge return-on-investment for both muscular power and cardiovascular conditioning. Start with small jumps (2-3 inches off the ground), and slowly progress to getting the feet higher off the ground or jumping on to a stable surface several inches high.

Begin standing with feet hip width distance apart. Sit down by dropping the rump low, getting the hips just below the knees, and bringing the elbows to inside the knees. Explode up, pressing the ground away, and lifting the body into the air. Once airborne, point the toes slightly to land on the balls of the foot. It is important to bend at three joints when squatting and landing - the ankle, knee, and hip. Try to land softly and under control.

Sumo Jump

The Sumo Jump is a variation of the squat jump that builds up flexibility and strength in the muscles that run along the inside of the thighs.

Start standing with a wide stance, feet pointing out at a 45 degree angle. Bend the knees and lower the rump down to touch the ground. Focus on maintains an upright back - do not hinge at the waist to touch the ground. Sit low and imagine sliding the back down a wall. After touching the ground, explode up and bring the feet together to touch. Immediately jump the feet back out into the sumo stance and lower back down, reaching for the ground. Complete one set of 10 repetitions.

Lunge Jump

The Lunge Jump challenges muscular power, cardiovascular conditioning, and coordination. Jumping and switching arms and legs in the air takes practice to execute the movement with control and fluidity.

Start standing and spewing back with the left leg. Drop the left knee close - but not touching! - the ground, creating a 90 degree angle with the front (right) leg. Explode upward and jump switch the legs in the air, driving the right leg back and the left leg forward. Land softly and lower into a lunge. Repeat. Complete one set of 10 repetitions per side.

Side Jump

Side Jumps strengthen the muscles on the outside of the legs, and build stability around the knee joint. Start with small jumps, covering just a few feet, to ensure that there is a controlled landing and that there is not excessive pressure put on the knees.

Start in a standing position. Stride the right leg out to the side and jump to land on the right foot. Allow the left leg to trail and tap the right foot. Immediately press off with the right foot and stride the left leg out to the side and jump to land on the left foot. Imagine ice skating or cross country skiing. Complete one set of 10 repetitions per side.

STRENGTH

Train movements, not muscles. Training muscles in isolation - working from a single joint (e.g. biceps curl) - creates incorrect motor programming and causes confusion for the muscles and the brain. This is because the muscles are asked to do one motion in training, then another motion in life. Muscles work together as part of an integrated unit; they should be trained in a similar manner.

Strength training is a means to an end, not an end itself. Start by developing healthy movement pattens using just bodyweight exercises (i.e. push ups, pull ups, air squats, toe touches). This will develop strength along with the balance, proprioception, and synergistic muscles needed to allow for proper progression and preparation for more challenging resistance.

Another great way to train functional strength is through movements that use multiple joints, in multiple planes of motion like working diagonally and rotationally. Using tools like kettlebells and dumbbells (or medium-sized rocks!) allow for these large, multidirectional/planar movements while working just one side of the body. This will simultaneously improve strength while challenging balanced and stabilization across the body.

Sets and Repetitions

Each week will have a different combination of sets and repetitions. For week one, the program is 5 sets of 10 repetitions. Complete 10 bodyweight squats. Rest for 30 seconds, then complete 10 push ups. Rest for 30 seconds, then complete 10 toe touches. Rest 30 seconds, then complete 10 rows. A round of squats, push ups, toe touches, and rows equals one set. Complete the same sequence four more times.

More or Less Challenging

All of the movements can be made more or less challenging. It is important to find the appropriate level for each movement.

Push ups, for example, can be made less challenging by elevating the hands. The least challenging is doing push ups with the hands on the wall. Lower the hands to progressively lower surfaces to identify the appropriate level. Progress from the wall, to a counter, to a coffee table, to the floor.

Need more of a challenge? Elevate the feet. Start by putting the feet on a stair. Progress up by elevating the feet to a chair.

<u>Squat</u>

The squat is a fundamental movement the is necessary to keep the body healthy, as well as maintain independence and free from movement aids like grab bars.

The human body needs to squat throughout the day to get in and out of chairs, up and down from the toilet, and in and out Fromm cars. Do not neglect squatting.

If it is too challenging to squat low and maintain proper form and balance, start by sitting down and rising up from a chair for support. Do not completely sit into the chair and lose the muscular tension in the legs, rather, let the rump "kiss" the chair and immediately rise back up to standing.

Start in a standing position with feet slightly wider than hip width distance apart. Begin to drop the rump and sit low. Imagine sliding the back down a wall. Sit down in between the knees, lowering the hips to just below knee height. Press back up by pushing the ground away through the center of the feet and return to standing tall. Complete all of the repetitions, rest 30 seconds, then complete the next movement.

Push Up

The Push Up is a classic strength move; a standard in fitness testing programs for decades. The Push Up is so much more than that, however. First, the name says it all. It is having the ability to get the body up - from a chair, the ground, etc. It is an essential human movement.

Those same pushing muscles are also used to open doors, push lawnmowers, and press carry-on luggage into the overhead compartment.

Start with the hands and feet on the floor in a push up position. Take a moment to check the alignment of the body. The shoulders should be down and away from the ears; the shoulder, elbow, and wrist should be in a straight line; the tailbone tucked and the muscles around the bellybutton feel switched on; the kneecaps are zipped up to engage the muscles in the thigh; the heel is directly over the ball of the foot.

Slowly lower the chest down to the ground, maintaining a straight line from the shoulders to the rump. Envision a stick (or better yet, use a real stick!) resting on the back of the head, the shoulder blades, along the spine,and down to the tailbone.

Have the elbow-shoulder-torso form a 45 degree angle as the body descends. Pause just above the ground and try to have the nose, chest, and bellybutton hover as close to the ground as possible without touching.

Press the body back up in a smooth and controlled manner. Avoid pressing the shoulder up and leaving the hips down, causing the torso to sag. If this happens, regress to a less challenging version by elevating the hands. If plank push ups are not challenging enough, progress to elevating the feet. Either way, maintain strict form to get the most from the movement.

Toe Touch

Toe Touches are one of the most underrated and overlooked human movements. Hinging at the waist is absolutely essential. Most people perform the movement throughout the day, and do so incorrectly, leading to back pain and muscle strains. Hinging at the waist is used to pick up laundry baskets and grocery bags. Make proper toe touches a priority and pain in the lower back melt away.

Toe Touches are a hip hinge, **not** a squat. Squats move the hips north and south. Toe Touches move the hips east and west. They are distinctly different movements.

To practice, start by standing 4-8 inches in front of a wall. Place the blade of an open hand against the hips. Press the rump back towards the wall and have the hips eat the hands, Pac-Man style. Keep pressing back until the rump "kisses" the wall. Then drive the hips forward and back to standing tall.

After practicing this movement and finding the proper movement pattern, repeat the same motion, but have the hands reach down towards the toes. Touching the toes in not required! Focus on maintaining proper form and lower the hands as far as possible without allowing the form to breakdown.

It is also important to keep the feet flat on the ground. Before starting the hinge motion, grab the ground with the toes and hold that grip throughout the entire movement. This will keep the feet engaged and improve balance.

Row

The Row, and most upper body pulling movements, can be challenging to practice. Not because they are difficult to complete, but because it is often challenging to find a stable surface to pull on. This is where the most creativity is needed. Do not skip pulling because it is challenging to find something to pull from! Rows and upper body pulls will have a major effect in shrinking the waistline and adding muscle to the torso.

Sturdy tables make a great option for rowing. Start by sitting on the ground under the edge of the table with the legs stretched out under the table. Firmly grasp the edge of the table and raise the hips up into a reverse plank. Hold this position for a moment and check that the abdomen is switched on and that there is a straight line from the heels to the hips. If this is too challenging, place the feet flat on the floor and keep the knees bent.

Slowly pull the chest up towards the table by engaging the large muscles in the back. Feel the shoulder blades pulling in towards the midline of the body. Squeeze them together at the top and pause before lowering back down under control. Maintain rigidity in the abdomen and keep the hip up; do not allow the hips to sag.

FROM ACORN TO MIGHTY OAK

What does it take to develop from a Mighty Acorn into a Mighty Oak? It takes consistent growth over a long period of time. This is the same process that a tiny acorn uses to grow into a hearty sapling and then into a robust tree. The process cannot be rushed. Be patient and take a long view. Do not focus on being healthy and active just for an upcoming vacation, rather, think about what it takes to be healthy and active over the age of 100.

How long until a healthy and active life is achieved? This will vary for each person. This is because everyone will be starting at a different level of health, have a different level of commitment, and a different definition of healthy. It is important to remember that health is not a destination - it is a way of life. Once a desired level of wellness is attained, it is necessary to continually maintain that level of wellness through consistent nutrition, movement, and recovery.

Seriously, how long? Ok, here is a general template. Most new healthy behaviors will get positive results for most people for about one month. Through proper nutrition movement and recovery, by day 6, the face will be less puffy and the body less sweaty. On day 12, pants will be less tight and the belly less bloated. Day 18 will have joints less creaky and shirts fitting less tight. By day 24, energy levels will be high throughout the day and friends will start to take notice and ask for the" secret."

Then what? That is when it will become more challenging. After the first month, making small changes will no longer yield large improvements. The health improvements will become more incremental. Be patient and stay the course.

After approximately six months of consistent dedication to nutrition, movement, and sleep, there will be noticeable, sustainable changes. The body will have reset. The brain will be more clear, energy will be consistently high all day, sleep will be deep and rejuvenating, body fat will be replaced by lean muscle, and mobility will be significantly improved. This is where many people think that the work is done and begin to coast. Just like the slow process to achieving health, the reverse is also true. People at this stage begin to slowly erode the healthy habits and slide back into doing the things that got them unhealthy in the first place. Do not get complacent! Remember: lifetime commitment, not a destination.

After approximately 2-3 years of being committed to a healthy and active lifestyle, most people will have broken through and are in for the long haul. If that sounds like a long time, again, widen the view. Start thinking in terms of decades, not months.

Do not get overwhelmed! While it is a long, slow process, stay focused on the immediate tasks. Do not get discouraged by small setbacks or unforeseen challenges. Again, take the long view. There will be moments of weakness at a breakfast buffet, or injuries from over-enthusiastic activities - that is ok! Maintain the long view and see the setbacks for what they are - a small blip on the journey to leading a healthy and active lifestyle.

THE MIGHTY OAK STRENGTH STANDARD

Before attempting to lift heavy weights, it is important to build relative strength - the ability to move one's body with ease and efficiency. Just like not all oak trees look identical with the same number of branches or leaves, becoming a Mighty Oak will vary from person-to-person. Below is an example of a Mighty Oak Athletic bodyweight workout. Complete the sequence without having to break the reps up to be a true Mighty Oak!

Reps	Movement
25	Pull Ups
50	Push Ups
50	Squats
20	Chin Ups
40	Feet Elevated Push Ups
40	Toe Touches
15	Close Grip Pull Ups
30	Hands Elevated Push Ups
30	Sumo Squats
10	Neutral Grip Pull Ups
20	Overhead Presses
20	Walking Lunges

NEXT STEPS TO STAY HEALTHY AND ACTIVE

Completed the Month 1 Training Program? Well done! Now is the time to keep the momentum going.

Free Weekly Newsletter

Start by subscribing to the FREE newsletter at <u>MightyOakAthletic.com</u> for weekly motivation, videos, and tips on nutrition, movement, and recovery.

Free Health Coaching Call

Schedule a FREE Health Coaching call to discuss the biggest health challenge and identify solutions for improving health and wellness.

Monthly Newsletter

Ready for the full health experience? Sign up for the paid newsletter at <u>**MightyOakAthletic.com**</u> to receive monthly training programs, strength and conditioning videos, mobility videos, healthy recipes, nutrition recommendations, and more!

13 for 30 Weight Loss Program

Need to lose weight? Checkout the Mighty Oak Athletic *13 Pounds in 30 Days Weight Loss Program*. The program does not require any special workout equipment. No fancy foods or tricky cooking techniques. No increased time working out or excessive training. No calorie restriction or starvation. All it takes to lose 13 pounds in 30 days is a commitment to take a walk every day, eat wholesome foods, and get plenty of sleep. Simple, right? Get the program and lose the weight!

Free t-shirt

Connect with Mighty Oak Athletic on social media for a chance to win free t-shirts, water bottles, and more! Share photos and videos with #MightyOakAthletic.

Facebook
@MightyOakAthletic

Instagram
@MightyOakAthletic

Pinterest
@MightyOakAthletic

Twitter
@MightyAthletic

Thank you becoming a part of the Mighty Oak Athletic community!

Learn to Live Healthy

MEET THE MIGHTY OAK

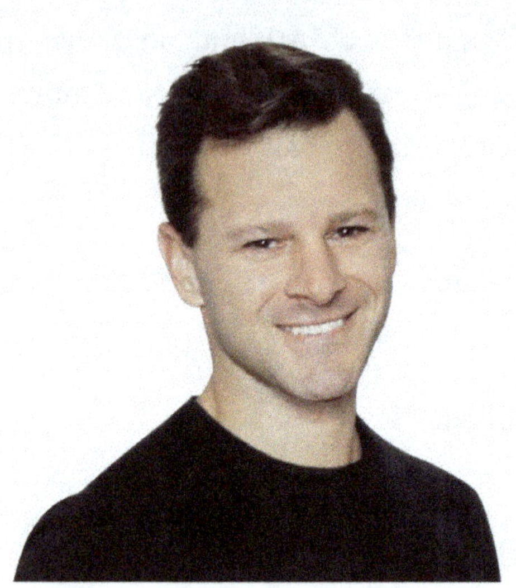

Michael Ockrim has been studying and practicing a healthy lifestyle for over 30 years. Excited to share the knowledge he has obtained, Michael earned a nationally-accredited health coaching certification and founded a health and wellness company, Mighty Oak Athletic.

Michael's passion is sharing how he has maintained a healthy lifestyle while raising four children, managing a career, enjoying hobbies, and even finding a few minutes to relax with his beautiful wife Carey.

www.ingramcontent.com/pod-product-compliance
Lightning Source LLC
Chambersburg PA
CBHW051810050726
47598CB00006B/2494

2

PARK BENCH NAP

NICE SUNNY DAY. I AM JUST WAITING for my usual customer. Should be coming about now. Yes - right on schedule.

Ah – down you go, easy, easy. I am getting older so please don't just plop down. Together we can ride 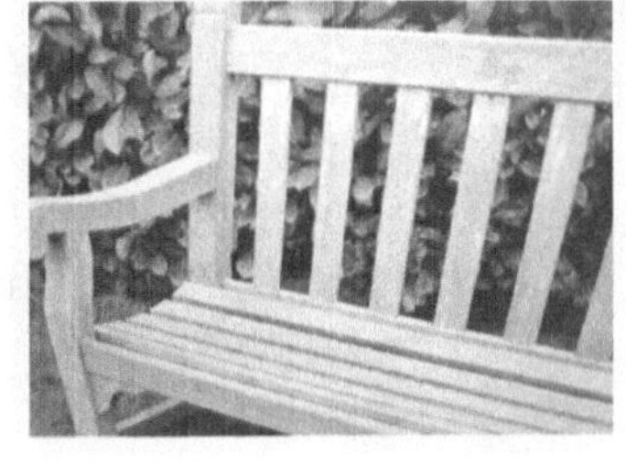 into the sunset if we take care of each other. Missed you yesterday. You mentioned something to that friend that stopped by a few days ago that you had an appointment. Did I hear correctly? Was it really that serious?

You know, I have been aging too. An occasional power wash and a fresh coat of paint but underneath it's still just me. I'm just like you except you can't cover up as good as I can. But we two are, never-the-less, getting older. Some things can't be hidden like your walk and talk. For me, it's holding you secure and bracing for the kids that sometimes run and jump when mom is not watching. Someday I just may give way. At my age, I don't think I will get repaired.

I know you and I have been seeing more and more of each other these last few years. It's been so nice to have you rest a while each day. I get to see the newspaper, smell those good pastry treats you have in the paper bag, and listen to the small talk you and your friends have as they walk by. Nothing really new most of the time, just friendly "have a nice day" stuff. That was, until a few days ago.

And there you go again. Starting to doze off for your afternoon snooze. I will hold you secure so go ahead and nap. Better wedge yourself against one of my arms, however. I know you need me so I will be strong for you. I get to see a lot of people but none as caring as you. You always clean up and never say a bad word. I can tell you appreciate me and the park. You always find me. I am your favorite bench. We are such good friends made just for each other.

Today your daughter came to take you home. Why is that? Will I see you tomorrow?

3

SHORT ON THE SIDES

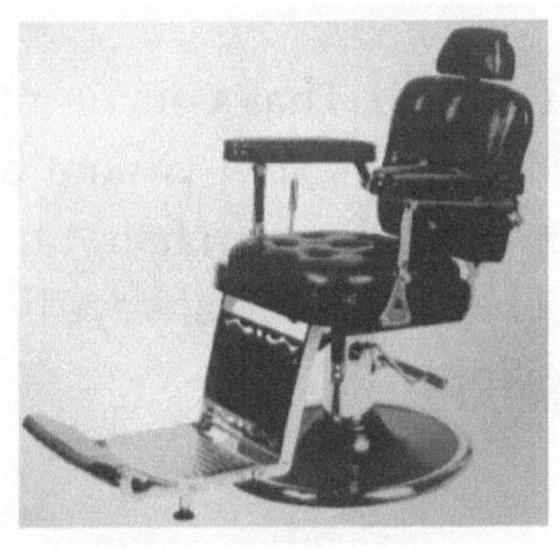

Come on in.

Boy, yesterday was a busy day. I hardly got time to get brushed off. Hope today is a little slower. Some reading material or TV to watch while you wait? Only one ahead in my chair so it shouldn't be too long.

I have a lot of customers, some young, some old. All have one thing in common. They need a haircut. But that is where the similarities end. How many opinions are there? Most want to look like someone else. Why not just look like yourself? I see you about every month, give or take a week or so. What will it be this time? Same as last? Shorter here, longer there? OK, let's get going. My chair is getting tired with you just sitting there.

I have some customers who have been life-long friends and I am more patient with them. But you are a newcomer and perhaps one of those quick-change types. No loyalty at all. Get a slightly bad cut and off to try another barber chair. Well today I will try to pretend we are friends. I will give you my soft seat that rotates and eases up and down. No special treatment. Everyone gets the same. We barber chairs have been a part of your life for a long time. You remember us very well. Locations change, but a chair is always there to do its job. We are sturdy and reliable. I can't do anything about the guy doing the cutting, however. You will just have to put up with all the chatter. Enjoy the TV. Be still and don't move.

Too bad we only have an occasional get together. We might be better friends if you could give me more time. I could tell you so many stories. The hair cutter only gives you a quick pass where I could get into the details. You see, I get close to the flesh, so to speak. So close I can feel your pulse and temperature, and even some sweat when the talk gets too close for comfort.

As soon as the cutting stops, up and off you go. That's ok, don't thank me. I am used to the same "no turn and exit" without a hint of gratitude for the time you spent in my barber chair. But remember, no matter where you go for a haircut, I will always be there for support. And that's the bottom line.

4

BEST BALLGAME SEAT

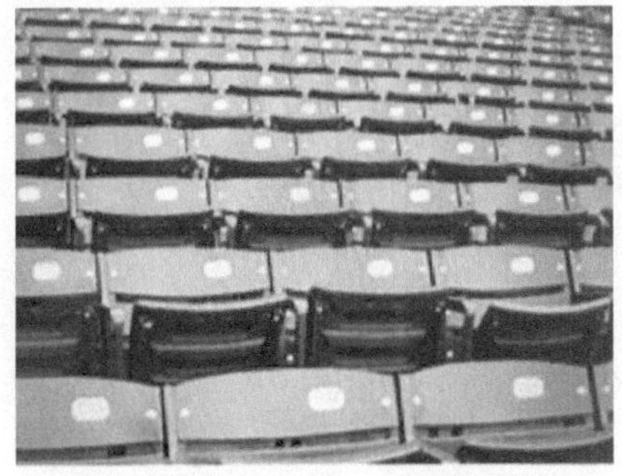

I just sit here most of the time. Well not actually sit. That's what you do. I am here to give you a place to sit on game days.

Look around and see some 40,000 or more just like me. I am lucky, I suppose, because I am a highly sought-after seat. Those seat guys in the upper decks and way down the lines and in dead center field only get action in big games and the 4th of July fireworks game. I'm row 20 and square with third base on the home team side. Everybody thinks I am the best.

You are the lucky one today. Season opener and a big crowd expected. You made it past the gates, inspection, and just had to buy a program with all the player pictures. You passed the food vendors but made quick mental note where your favorites are for later.

We go through the whole getting acquainted routine again. I hear you double checking your ticket stubs and discussing what you can see, where the concession stands are, parking, stairs, rest rooms, etc. And perhaps the most important, what your neighbors are like. Yes, you learned the unwritten ballpark etiquette from an early age going with dad and mom. But times are changing and each year slight changes try to pry themselves into the rule book. Take for example that annoying wave thing. Where did that come from? Who let it into the acceptable routine? And every so often it gets quite uncomfortable with too much beer and some bad manners, irritable yelling, and standing to block your view. But thank goodness this is the exception and most of the old standards still remain. I think today will be a fine day for baseball.

I see you have your glove today. I have been here since the park opened and don't remember ever seeing a foul ball land on my seat. A ricochet or two came close last year but no luck. There is always a first so keep that glove ready for action. Hot dogs already? It's only the second inning. Peanuts, sodas, and nachos? Hey—when did nachos get in the play book? Every inning there is an isle vendor to contend with, yelling, "Beer here! Pass this down!" Part of the game, I guess. Can we just sit still a while?

Time goes slowly. Don't you know it had to be a pitcher's duel today! You wanted to see a home run, but all we get to see are ground outs. Oh well, defense is exciting too, you try to convince yourself. Yes, I know my seat is starting to get quite firm on your posterior. Just wait to the seventh inning stretch where you get to stand up and chant, "root, root, root for the home team," or excuse yourself for the restroom.

Time for the big decision. I know you well. It happens just about now in every game. Should you stay, or leave? Go now and beat the traffic? No, it's a close game, so you decide to stay.

Last out! Finally, working your way out with the late crowd, you reflect. What a time you had—no matter the score. Nothing like a good seat at the old ballgame.

5

———————————

GREEN PEAS

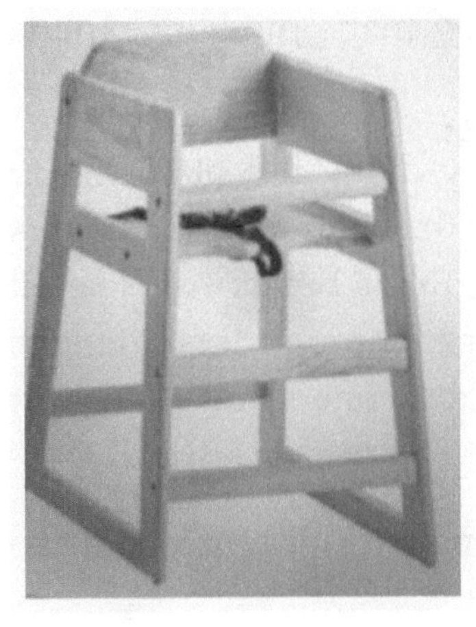

I'M THE CHAIR THAT HAS TO PUT UP with a lot. Kids either love my highchair or can't stand to be in me. And it seems to vary each time. You never know what it will be. I try my best not to complain.

I know you appreciate what I do. So, let's have lunch.

You got me used from your sister for a fraction of my new price. Boy, was that a job with her two! Glad that job is over. I was new back then, but like a new car, one meal and I was quickly broken in and depreciated. But I learned a lot, so I am ready for action again. The little ones are so cute until the food doesn't go where it is supposed to go. On the floor, on fingers, on you, and that's just the first spoonful. Oh no, peas again. I hate that mushy green stuff. It goes everywhere, even under the tray. Talk about a cleanup challenge.

Apple sauce is a little stickier, but it just smells better and is sweeter. I'd rather clean it up any day off those rosy little cheeks.

Do you know I was made in a baby furniture factory? I started out as just a bunch of lumber, some metal, and assorted hardware. At one point I was going to get into the baby crib production line and then got switched to highchairs at the last minute. I guess I get all the luck. No, I'm not complaining. You seem to know what you are doing. I'm hoping these next few months go smoothly. But still, I just can't stop thinking what life would have been like being the crib and sleeping most of the time versus having to be ready for action, mess, and cleanup several times each day.

Lunch over? Not sure? Try another spoonful? Try some cheerios for a distraction while you attend to the phone. Yes, that is a challenge, but now you know why they made mothers experts at multi-tasking.

Hey, you can really scrub. Go easy. Try doing it a little sooner before the green peas dry. Don't forget those little messy fingers went a lot of places during lunch. Ah, that's better. All cleaned and ready for another meal. We can get through this. You are well on your way to training good table manners and I can start planning for retirement.

What did you say? Your sister wants me back? There's going to be another?

There goes my retirement.

6

YOU BE THE JUDGE

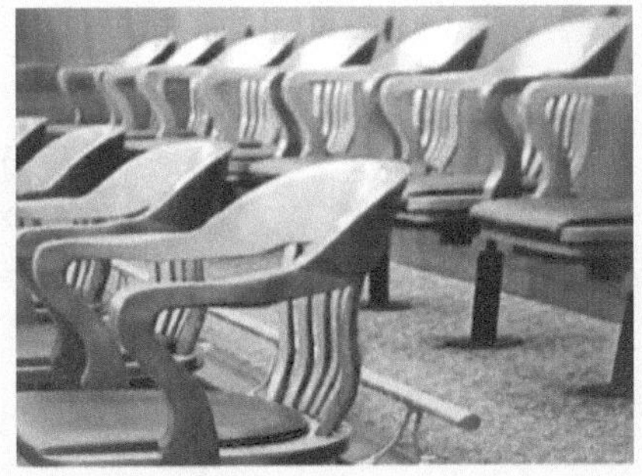

Here they come. 12 new ones. Just the same routine, however.

Is this your first jury? Well good for you doing your duty. Go ahead and take my seat. Yes, right here. They are all alike. Many before you have sat where you are. I bet you will be just as nervous and uncertain. The only solace is you get to be here, and not out there. I will hold you firm. Go ahead and grasp my arms for more security.

But you have not yet passed the tests so don't claim this chair as your own quite yet. Both sides get to find out if you can help or might hurt their client. They will ask you all kinds of questions. Some are easy to understand why, but others seem very obscure. You probably won't figure out why. Answer truthfully and honestly. If I don't see you again, it's been nice knowing you.

Well, you made it. Now pay attention. There will be all kinds of instructions. And when the attorneys start talking they may be looking right at you. Yes, I know. One has already done this to every one of you. Made you very uncomfortable, didn't it? You felt like sinking lower in my chair if I would let you. You know you are supposed to be impartial. Then why was that attorney seeming to make you a friend I hear you thinking to yourself. You are learning fast. Keep a straight face, no emotion or body shifting.

Hours, days, how long has it been setting in my chair? Finally, the judge instructs you to rise and exit to the jury room for deliberation. That's what they call it, but it will probably be a bunch of arguing. When I see you again it will only be brief. You will sit in my chair, you and me, for the last time.

What fate will you impart?

It may seem like you have been on trial.

In the end you had to vote, perhaps still uncertain as when we first met?

7

SWING A WHILE

I'm always here. Me and the porch. A lovely place.

Who will come and sit a while this early evening? Will it be the little ones all giggly and wiggly? Or maybe mom and dad to review the day? Or even the young teens 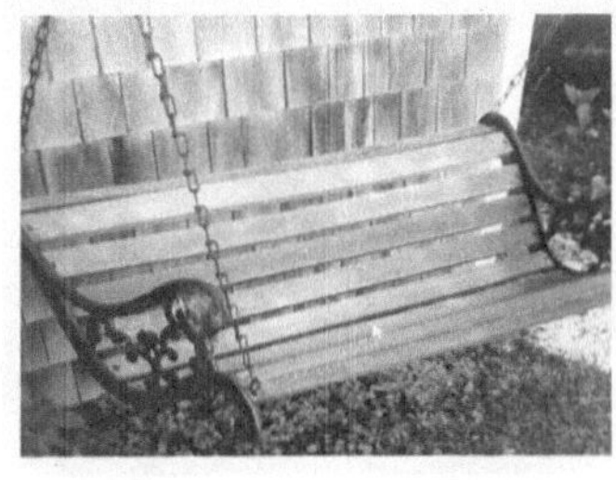 all full of the future? So many, and yet I am still the same old swing.

Oh yes, I forgot, you old folks. The ones that appreciate me the most. The ones who have been through all the years. Come and swing one more time this evening. You decide what to talk about. I hope it's not about the latest aches and pains. I have them too but would rather hear you remember the good times when anything was possible. You can't do it over, but you can tell what it was like. Yes, I know, each telling gets a little vaguer, some parts forgotten, and events perhaps recast a bit. But that is the pleasure of hearing you share it with each other. You need your memory journeys to make sense of everything.

Sometimes as the time passes the conversation gives way to just listening to the evening sounds and watching the day say good-night. So peaceful and soothing. Getting slightly cooler and just a hint of a breeze. I enjoy our visits. I can still give all of you what you need. Just remember, I need care too. Take it easy, better to just swing me easy these days. I seem to be developing a squeak somewhere on my chain. I hear you saying, "gotta put a little oil on that." Good news for my old chains. But if you don't get around to it, I'll understand.

Last swing tonight? Will we get together tomorrow?

I know the answer. You know it too.

Porch light out.

8

MIDDLE SEAT

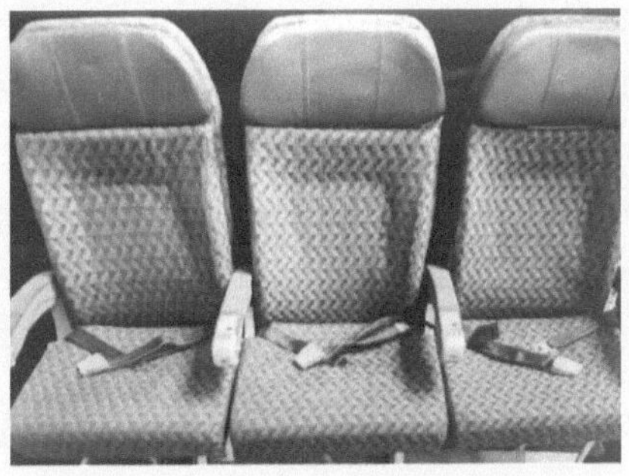

HOW WOULD YOU LIKE TO BE THE LEAST LIKED SEAT ON THE PLANE?

I never asked for this assignment. Why, why, why?

All us seats started out to be an important part of the exciting airline business. Yes, flying to faraway places with customers excited to be traveling. But when it became time for seat installation, I got shoved into the middle between two friends I went through the production line with.

Initially I tried to make the best of it. I smiled and held a firm back. But as the passengers came, flight after flight, I got the same repeated comments. Some were loud but most just low volume disgruntled one-liners about getting stuck with the middle seat. Once in a while we have even had near fights over who has to sit on me.

Now, just being the middle seat is not all to the story. You passengers have a never-ending string of complaints. I know they keep sliding our rows inches or fractions closer for an additional row of passengers or to just add it to a few rows up front to charge a "more leg room" premium. But for you back in coach it results in less leg room and more difficulty getting out to the restrooms.

Now consider those few more inches you keep adding. Don't you have to take some blame for the crowding? On the positive side, we have even been redesigned to be slimmer to help recover some space. But I have to admit we have less padding and that makes those long flights a little more uncomfortable. But again, we have tried to make up for this inconvenience with enhanced electronic connections and controls built into our arms rests for your technical device enjoyment. Always thinking of our guests.

You say you can't put the tray down like you used to?

Well, suck it in a bit. As I mentioned, part of this tight fit is your fault.

Who needs a tray these days anyway? Notice the lack of meals and snacks?

Say something nice about my middle seat next time.

I'll try and put up with you too.

9

THE COUCH NEEDS LOVE

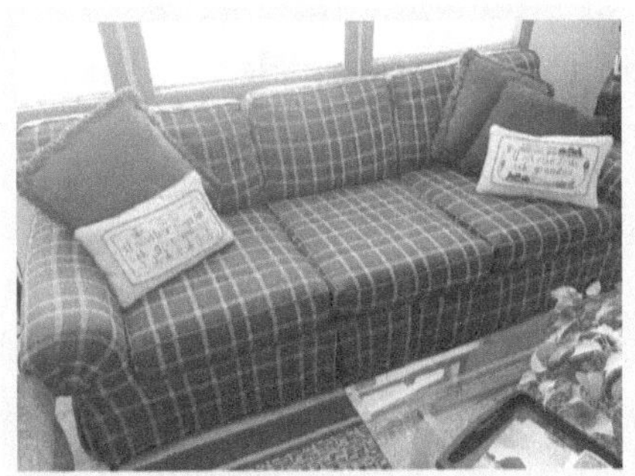

I NEED RESPECT, TOO.

Yes, more respect than you normally give something you sit on. I get most of the longer-term sitters and even those afternoon naps and occasional overnight stays. So, you see, I get a lot of use those ordinary chairs don't.

Now, I am not asking for any medals or awards. Just a little recognition for the job I do. And unlike a chair I have accommodated you in all kinds of moods. All the way from just plain worn out to snuggling in for a favorite TV show. Even the popcorn you drop down my cracks doesn't offend me. Just tell me you're sorry and will clean it up later.

But no, I'm afraid that last thing I mentioned does not happen very often. Only when company is coming over do you pull up my cushions and vacuum what you left last month, things too embarrassing to mention here. I only get special treatment when my shabby appearance is about to reflect on you. Adding "designer" pillows and small throws are only further insults to my purpose.

So, naturally, I am just a little upset.

Now that I am all clean and neat, let's see if I can stay that way. Can we at least give it a try? It just takes a little more caring. What about a "no eating on the couch" policy? Remember, you tried that in the car after something similar happened there. Yes, I know it did not last long but at least you tried. That's all I'm asking. Give it a try.

Whatever happens, I will be just as soft and comforting as before. You and the dog, the kids, and even mom can relax in just about any position you wish. I will try to hold you and all of them and not complain. You can play games, watch TV, have a party, or just do nothing. Doesn't matter to me. Only one thing. When you and mom are out, the kids sometimes get a little crazy. "King of the couch" seems to be a favorite sport, but my springs really take a pounding.

And the last thing. When no one is home the dog gently hops up, sniffles for a good spot, circles once or twice, and settles down on me so smooth, hardly making a dent.

If only people were dogs. They love me more.

AFTERWORD: IF THEY HAD A VOICE

Have you ever wondered what our world has to say?

We go about our lives midst all forms of non-human objects with only a passing thought, or no thought at all about them. And rarely have we even attempted a conversation.

What if we listen closely? What would they tell us? What could we learn?

You might be surprised at just how much they have to say about us.

This series of short stories started by an impromptu response to a prompt given in a writing class I took. The prompt was to write for 14 minutes on "something you keep." Out of the blue the image of a beach rock in my hand came to mind. Probably from one of many walks on the beach at Cape Meares, and even seeing others looking for that special rock. Or even seeing someone's beach and shell collection neatly arranged or scattered around. We all have picked up a beach rock, held it a while, and maybe kept it to go home or dropped it for another. That day I wrote about this experience, completed the assignment, and filed it away with that hint of something undone.

Several months later as I was typing my handwritten responses to past writing prompts into the computer, I again read the story I had titled, "The Hopeful Beach Rock." I lingered a while, reading it again several times. And for some mysterious reason the stories started coming one after the other about other beach objects like driftwood, waves, the ocean breeze, and more. All had something to say about us. They even ask questions and heard our thoughts. They started our memories working and recalling earlier times, ones that were happy, sad, and adventurous.

After doing several beach stories I started to get images of other things we pass by, touch, or work with that should also get a chance to talk. Thus, started a much larger series of stories including things we sit on, doors we go through, and a range of others you will want to read about in the Voices collections.

This is the best part. I realized that in telling these as short stories, some call flash fiction, I could give you the chance to make it your own. I give each a range of emotions and experiences, but you will find it compelling to fill in and expand with your own.

As you read the stories remember only the non-human object does the talking. You have only to listen. The chair, for example, will ask you to remember what you were doing and thinking as you sat for a while, then suggests answers and asks even more questions. The door will recall memories of your emotions the door had observed as you passed through. Like a mirror, the door reflects these and suggests what you were thinking and whether you had any regrets. The beach rock wonders and asks you if you will keep it or discard it and choose another leaving you to determine the outcome. Interesting life lessons for sure.

Each reader of these stories will have a unique reaction to the observations and answers to the questions because all have different experiences. The one common link is we all have these kinds of memories. And each subsequent reading will only add to the recall and variations, with even new themes and outcomes of your own.

Some stories were written on the lighter side of things, playful, and happy times. Some are more serious with only hints of deeper concerns, but none are scary or tragic. Some have a moral bent and others suggest you read between the lines to get the nuance.

Most stories, however, are just plain fun.

ABOUT THE AUTHOR

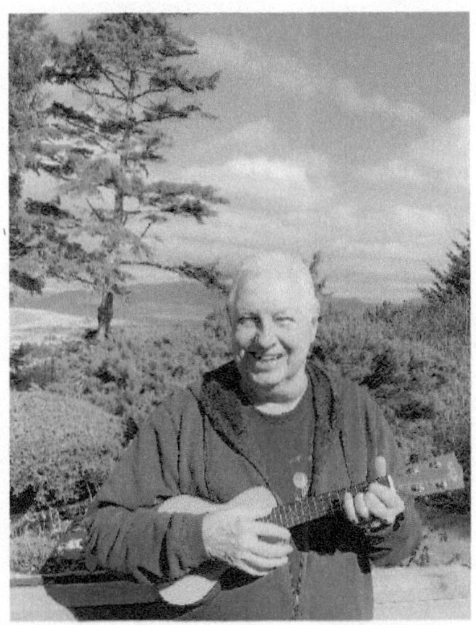

I give most of the inspiration credit to the wonderful Northwest and Oregon coast. I arrived in 2015 and have not stopped creating in new and unusual ways. It inspires all art forms, and frankly just about anything you want to do. So, I give thanks for a second chance to prosper including my efforts of fiction writing and just recently song writing.

After a first degree in Fine Arts from California State University I went into business for my professional life. An MBA from the University of Denver followed while working for three major US companies, then running and starting my own along the way.

Concurrent to the business side I was an adjunct professor in the MBA program for the University of Phoenix for over 30 years.

I guess I was destined to return to the creative side of life, now at the ripe old age of 81. Old dogs, new tricks? Perhaps in this case. Yes, this is not your typical "about the author?" Blame the weather.

VOICES PUBLICATION COLLECTION

Beach Voices

Doors We Walk Through

The Chair Has Something To Say

Walk In My Garden

What's In The Box

Clothes Get Testy

Food Talks Back

ALSO BY BRAD AYERS

A Life's Journey

Beach Voices

www.ingramcontent.com/pod-product-compliance
Lightning Source LLC
Chambersburg PA
CBHW021349060726
47591CB00006B/2227